The Beat Your
**Body Chaos** Diet

MONICA GRENFELL

# The Beat Your
## Body Chaos Diet

PAN BOOKS

First published 2001 by Pan Books
an imprint of Macmillan Publishers Ltd
25 Eccleston Place, London SW1W 9NF
Basingstoke and Oxford
Associated companies throughout the world
www.macmillan.com

ISBN 0 330 48151 7

9 8 7 6 5 4 3 2 1

A CIP catalogue record for this book is available from
the British Library.

Typeset by SX Composing DTP, Rayleigh, Essex
Printed and bound in Great Britain by
Mackays of Chatham plc, Chatham, Kent

To Michael, for all his patience

# Contents

Acknowledgements                                                    xi
Introduction                                                       xiii


## Body Chaos                                                        1

### Chapter One  **What is Body Chaos?**                             3

What To Do When 'Nothing Works'                                      6
Hellish Hormones                                                     7
Heavenly Hormones                                                    8
Turning to the Experts                                               9
All In the Same Boat                                                10
Back to Nature                                                      11
Mental Attitude                                                     12
What's Food Got To Do With It?                                      13
Your Best Friend                                                    15
Here's What I'll Be Looking At In This Book                         15
My Mission                                                          17
Mental Chaos                                                        19

### Chapter Two  **Hormones**                                       25

The Hormones Common To Us All                                       26
A Day In the Life of Your Hormones                                  41
Your Uniquely Female Hormones                                       43
Hormone Hell                                                        62

## Chapter Three **Allergies and Additives** — 72

Too Many Additives — 73
Allergies and Sensitivities — 76
Keeping a Food Diary — 79
Your Polluted Body! — 82

## Chapter Four **What Is Your Body Made Of?** — 85

Fat — 86
Muscle — 89
Bones — 90

## Chapter Five **It Must Be In My Genes!** — 92

Is It Wrong to Encourage Dieting? — 95
Stop Weighing Yourself All the Time!' — 96
What Am I Doing Wrong? — 100
Can't be Bothered? — 101

## Chapter Six **Eating Your Way Out of Chaos** — 103

Getting Started With the Right Diet — 103
What You Need In a Good Diet — 106
The Way to Lose Weight — 121
Dying to be Slim – When Dieting Turns Ugly — 126
The Miracle of Homeostasis and Leptin — 129
Your Body – Giving It the Final Word — 136

# Beat Your **Body Chaos** 137

## Chapter Seven **Mental Attitude** 139

The Benefits of Routine 142
All In the Mind 144
Mental Gremlins 149
The Good News About Adopting New Eating
  Habits 153
Realistic Expectations 154
Keeping Pace With Your Changing Metabolism 157
Some of Your Excuses for Giving Up 158

## Chapter Eight **Before Your Weight-Loss Plan** 170

Your Basic Daily Calorie Requirements 170
Energy Balance 171
I Don't Know Where to Start 174
Planning Your Meals 176
Eating Habits 177
Improve Your General Health 179

## Chapter Nine **So What do I Have to Eat?** 185

The BEAT YOUR BODY CHAOS Diet 187
Water Retention Prevention Diet 204
Sensible Wheat-free Diet 210
Good Mood Diet – Anti-stress, Anxiety and Depression 218
Teen Chaos Diet 223
Pre-menstrual Body Chaos Diet 229
Pregnancy Chaos Diet 239
Mid-life Chaos Diet 246
Weight-Gain Diet 253

Chapter Ten **Exercise: I want to look Gorgeous**                    255

Never Too Late                                                      259
Finding Time                                                        260
Can I Reclaim my Lost Muscles?                                      262
Common Myths                                                        263
Exercise and Your Heart                                             263
Exercise and Appetite                                               263
The Psychological Benefits of Exercise                              266
Exercise and Endorphins                                             266
Insulin Sensitivity                                                 268
Starting Young                                                      268
Exercise in Your Teens                                              269
Exercise in Your Twenties and Thirties                             270
Exercise and Pregnancy                                             270
Stopping the Clock                                                  271
Exercise in Your Forties and Fifties                               272
Your Plan of Action                                                 272
To Conclude                                                         273

Chapter Eleven **Recipes**                                          274

**Finally**                                                         293

**Food File**                                                       294

Carbohydrate and Sugar Guide                                        294
Proteins                                                            300
Glycaemic Index                                                     304

# Acknowledgements

I am grateful to the following people for their assistance with this book and for their help in untangling for me all the technical details:

Dr Beverley Carey, MBBS BSc
Centre for Nutritional Medicine

Dr Adam Carey, MSc MB BCht MA MRCOG
Centre for Nutritional Medicine

Professor John Garrow, MD PhD FRCP

Dr Roger Chapman, MD BSc MBBS FRCP
Radcliffe Hospital, Oxford

Miss Clair Flynn, Chartered Physiotherapist

# Introduction

I have been a diet and fitness writer and a journalist for many years, and have spent much of my time solving the problems of thousands of readers who write to me about their weight and figure problems. But the wonderful thing about the letters I receive is that they tell a complete story. For example, a woman might write to complain about the shape of her legs, but she will start her letter by saying, 'I am married for the second time, I have two children of my own and two stepchildren and my husband is currently unemployed.' She might go on to describe an operation she has had, her moods, their lack of money and along the way refer back to her legs. Another correspondent might say 'I have everything I could ever want or need, a fabulous career and no money worries, but the state of my body when I was on the beach recently made me want to curl up and die.' So you see, I get the complete picture of their lives.

Two threads run through all these problem letters which unite their writers in a common purpose: they want to feel in control of their bodies and they want to feel good about their appearance.

Many women let themselves go, that is clear. It is also their right. 'Letting go' does not necessarily mean looking a mess, being scruffy and getting fat, it can mean simply letting go of the tensions which have kept you to a certain standard. Deciding to shift the standards in one area of your life in order to devote time to another is a sensible decision which suggests time and priority management and is to be admired. But letting yourself go because you have tried and failed to conquer something you feel should be eminently conquerable is depressing and frustrating.

Not being able to stick to a diet is one thing, but sticking to a diet and not achieving anything is quite another. 'Where am I going wrong?' is a phrase I have seen written in more letters than there are days in a lifetime. People feel that far from living an unhealthy, unfit life, they are doing all they can to maintain their shape, health and looks, but nothing is working. In this book I have set out to give you a superb, healthy, hormone-friendly, weight-loss diet and to answer most of your questions about why you feel so bad, why your body won't do what you want it to do, and why you're in chaos.

I hope it is a comfort to you to know that I am not some young fitness expert who cannot understand why everybody does not have my fantastic energy and good health. It is dispiriting to see such young women bouncing about and delivering lectures on how to feel bright and breezy and have a fantastic figure. I can tell you that most of what I write about in this book I have experienced myself. I have been through all three stages of the female experience described in this book, which does not cover the very senior age group, and I overcame them because I had to, or go mad. I suppose you could say that this was the book I looked for then and couldn't find.

The inspiration for the title of this book came from a wonderful young endocrinologist called Beverley Carey. She was not my doctor, but circumstances forced us together for ten minutes and the idea for this book was conceived. I am forever in her debt.

# Body Chaos

# Chapter One

# What is Body Chaos?

Do you ever wake in the morning, remember what your body looks like and feel your heart sink? Is it so long since you felt really well that you can't actually remember it? Does the doctor draw a blank, or prescribe the first thing that seems to fit the bill? It's demoralizing to feel that nobody in the world understands your problem, that you're a freak who's doing something wrong. This is body chaos. It happens when, despite your heroic efforts to the contrary, your body does its own thing, but don't worry – you're going to overcome it.

Being in chaos is, of course, totally subjective: your idea of a vaguely off day might have someone else reaching for the tranquillizers; your weight neurosis may have another person scratching their head in disbelief. Nor is it fair that your stomach is always bloated because you suffer from chronic water retention for at least half the month. But fairness has nothing to do with it. It's sometimes hard to accept that hormones are the primary cause of this nightmare. You may think your chaos is caused by outside influences – that it's your overbearing mother-in-law or hyperactive office assistant who drive you to such distraction. You reason that your weight gain isn't your fault, that you over-eat out of anxiety, or are so busy at work you haven't time for exercise. But in reality the driving force behind all your body processes are your hormones, and in this book I am going to help you to get a grip on them, rebuild yourself with their help and turn the entire situation to your advantage.

Age is a funny thing. Take sixteen. Is it young? Not to a child of eight. Even if you're middle-aged you're still a girl to the pensioner next door. So our concept of age needs perspective, and body chaos comes into play when things happen to us which we're not ready for. We think in terms of huge chunks of, or leaps in, age. When we're fifteen we look to the age of twenty as the next milestone in life; at twenty you're thinking 'when I'm thirty . . .'

I was reminded of this when I heard a famous Hollywood actress being interviewed the other day. She was about to have her fortieth birthday, and the interviewer asked her how she felt about this, given that she had been associated in the past with young 'bimbo' acting roles. 'It's quite scary,' she replied, 'but I'm looking forward to it. I don't really know how it's going to feel, so I'll take it one day at a time.' But I wonder what she was expecting? Turning forty happens in a matter of twenty-four hours as for any other day. Her attitude put me in mind of school. You get to the final year of one school and emerge one of the eldest, most confident, swaggering and self-important students, then hey presto! you start the next school six weeks later and become one of the youngest students, ill at ease, nervous and insecure. You are the same person as before but people look at you differently and so you feel different. It happens again when you leave school for university and it goes on throughout life: from the top of one hill you go to the foot of the next one.

So is getting older like this? Is a teenager secretly thinking that being twenty will be her passport to adulthood? Perhaps that fortieth birthday is seen as a kind of promotion? But your body doesn't stand still for the years in between the milestones. Living-related changes are going on continually, and the first time you notice them is when you suddenly find that your weight has risen or you spot a patch of cellulite. It's like having your cut just a bit shorter than you wanted it, so short that you study yourself in the mirror every day to see if it has grown. That vital centimetre won't show for a couple of months, but, of course, just because you can't see your hair growing doesn't mean it isn't happening.

If only you could feel the same way about the effort you put into losing weight or getting a certain part of you in shape! Your cells are growing, dividing and dying all the time, and we all know that diseases like cancer or heart disease can take many years to develop – like a time bomb ticking away inside you when all the time you are feeling well and going about your daily business with vigour. So here you are quietly thinking that you can eat what you like, smoke and take no exercise and you're not worried about the effect on your health because you look fine. Then people write to me and say, 'The minute I turned fifty I gained a stone!' or, 'I've exercised like mad for six weeks and nothing's happened!' You see, just like the hair analogy, two factors come into play here: you don't notice the gradual changes in yourself as much as somebody else would and, although it takes time to see a difference, it would be impossible to imagine that once you've started an exercise programme absolutely nothing had changed about your body. It's simply not possible. So, the first rule of body management is to anticipate the changes, and the second rule is to be patient!

Because we tend to think of our lives in terms of leaps or stages, we believe that between these markers nothing happens: that you are born and somehow stay static until you leave home, then you are suddenly an adult. Reaching thirty or becoming a mother are hurdles which are not just life events, they put us into a different social category, rather as becoming a married woman used to signify maturity. But getting older is an ongoing process. Although we know that we get older, we rarely think we are going in that direction every day, so we say that we'll cross that bridge when we come to it. You believe that you stay the same at eighteen or twenty-five or whatever your favourite age is, and either you don't accept, or you ignore, the increasing signs of ageing until you've got a disaster on your hands and you're saving up for cosmetic surgery.

This is your body and nobody can look after it for you. Your mother isn't going to be there reminding you to do things for the rest of your life, or putting meals in front of you. It's down to you.


## What To Do When 'Nothing Works'

Unfortunately, a lot of women write to me to say that they've started their new exercise regime and diet plan full of optimism and high motivation, and they've followed my advice about being patient, but after a few weeks they still can't see a difference. Naturally they feel that if they're going to look the same with or without all the effort, expense and time, they might as well save themselves the trouble. I can quite see their point of view, and it's true to say that some-times I meet someone who has been on one plan or another for more than a year and who looks exactly the same as when she started. That's fine if you wanted to maintain a certain figure which you've already achieved, but if you're trying to shape up and lose a few kilos and you've not even lost one, something is indeed wrong. Haven't you ever been to the doctor, say for a skin problem, been given some cream which didn't work, and gone back to ask for something else? You might have had an infection which didn't respond to the particular antibiotics the doctor prescribed. Obviously they have worked for others so it wasn't a case of their being completely ineffective, only ineffective for you. It's the same for dieting and exercise; what works for one person doesn't necessarily work for another. When you're dealing with human beings rather than machines, you sometimes have to fine tune a bit.

## Hellish Hormones

Current thinking on women's life stages is hopelessly outdated, with new mothers still thought of as 'young' and menopausal women portrayed as silver-haired and having to be educated in the importance of exercise. The fact that half the new mothers these days are probably menopausal, and menopausal women are likely to have been doing aerobics for twenty years and be fitter than their daughters seems to have escaped most of the medical profession and advertising copywriters. Hormonal problems are a fact of life for us all and with a life expectancy of near-on eighty years these days, you could be looking at more than forty years of misery if you don't take steps to master those hormones. Doctors can give you wonderful pills and patches and devices to help, but it's not their job to try and explore your yo-yo weight gain. Your life can be successful in almost every other respect, but while everyone is enjoying themselves in all the latest outfits, you're covering up your arms, hiding your awful legs, sweltering in clothes you loathe and choosing the restaurant table nearest the door in case you get a panic attack.

This book is all about body chaos: right now your weight might be up and down, your hormones are raging, you have panic attacks and to cap it all you're having sleepless nights and hot flushes. Oh yes, didn't you know that the menopause doesn't start at fifty, it ends at fifty? The gradual winding down to middle age starts in your thirties, but nobody ever tells you the facts. Well I'm telling you, and a lot more besides.

I have spent over twenty-five years working in the fields of diet and nutrition, and I have written books and newspaper columns on the subject for over a decade. I know the misery that most women go through and my mailbag bulges every week with letters telling me about it. As a nutritionist I know that you can harness those hormones and rebuild yourself with their help.

## Heavenly Hormones

Hormones aren't only hell, they can be heavenly. It's easy to forget that there's a bright side to all this, whether it's the adrenalin rush you get when you're on a scary theme-park ride, the sexy, middle-of-the-month feeling which bathes you in a glow of self-confidence or the fabulous skin, hair and nails you get during pregnancy. Feeling and looking good are not just determined by how the dice fall, you *are* in control. Your body is simply an engine room, a powerhouse which feeds those hormones and helps them to perform well. Tiredness can be tamed with a diet which balances out the glycaemic index of carbohydrates so you feel energetic all the time. Hot flushes can be helped by a diet rich in phytoestrogens (plant oestrogens), anxiety can be calmed with food rich in the amino acid tyrosine and last but not least, your weight can be controlled not just by restricting calories, but by calming the impulses to binge.

You want to be quick off the mark, right as rain and raring to go, and I will explain how to go about this as the book progresses. It's a challenge for me, well worth the effort for you, and all that matters is that you want to be happy and not let your life slip away in a haze of anger and bitterness about your body.

## Turning to the Experts

If you want to know how to run a successful business, you don't ask a bankrupt. The real experts in the body chaos story are the women who have been successful with their looks and appearance. I have always been fascinated by the fact that clinics and special centres for women's problems only study the people who are having difficulties. I know they do this because I asked them. Why not ask the women who have never gained or lost an ounce of weight how they do it? Why not ask someone who has never experienced premenstrual food cravings, how she lives and what she eats? In the course of my research for this book I decided to do just that. I talked to hundreds of women from all walks of life and all age groups, and discovered that being a woman is not an inevitable roller coaster of misery. Many women go from adolescence to old age without missing a beat, and it was to them that I turned when I wanted some answers. I was looking for a common thread and I found one. Could you really be the same weight at sixty as you were at sixteen, without depriving yourself? Was it possible not to have a single day of fatigue or sleeplessness, irritability or weight gain? Were they simply lucky? I don't believe that there is such a thing as luck in human metabolism, and I soon found my answer in the daily diaries I asked my volunteers to complete. Although I had suspected as much, I was still amazed at the similarity of their stories. In all cases, their routines and food preferences matched, and the order of their lives was remarkably similar. If ever there was a case for mastering your hormones through diet, this was it.

Hormones are intangible. You can't see them, yet they are as much a part of your body as the working parts. They can cause many problems such as diabetes, infertility or thyroid disease, but most women will sail through life, mercifully, without experiencing any of these problems. It is the smaller hormone fluctuations we all suffer which cause the most havoc. For most of us the general rule is that periods happen about thirteen times a year for about forty years, you'll probably have a baby and the menopause is inescapable. However, if hormonal problems were just a matter of coping with a few headaches, tiredness and water retention I wouldn't have a job, because you'd be off to your doctor for a few pills or you'd cope like you do with periods. It's not so much the hormones, as what they make us look like that tips us over the edge. Weight gain and bloatedness are bad enough on their own, but when they threaten to ruin a special event because you look so washed out and fat, it's a different ball game.

## All In the Same Boat

To cheer you up for a minute, at least hormones and body chaos know no boundaries of class or social status. You can get fat legs however rich you are. Just as a top-of-the-range, custom-built limousine outclasses the run-of-the-mill banger in all departments, run out of petrol or get a puncture and the outcome is the same. Hormones don't know you're wealthy. I have had many a well-heeled client confess to envying her housekeeper's trim figure or sleek legs, and paying vast sums for gym memberships or a personal trainer doesn't make the exercise any easier! Your sex hormones have one objective, and that is to put you in the best possible condition for breeding, meaning you need good stores of fat on those hips, buttocks and stomachs. It might not seem very cheering right now, but I can promise you that we're all in the same boat!

## Back to Nature

We are unique in the animal kingdom for having feelings and emotions rather than just reactions and instincts, but depression and anxiety are the price we have to pay. We take on too much, we get stressed, we worry about performing well and we fall in love. If a tiger loses out on a kill it sees the sense in walking away unembarrassed. Birds which quarrel in the day for territory, huddle together at night for warmth. By contrast, humans are swayed by emotions, we're stubborn, jealous and have to prove a point. This incredible psychological effort robs our bodies of reserves. We either eat too much, starve ourselves or let ourselves go because of stress, and very soon there's a disaster on our hands as the mental chaos sets in. You hate yourself, you worry about the future and your health goes haywire.

Animals don't worry about eating too much or getting fat; they have no tussles with their consciences over second helpings. They have no aesthetic appreciation of their appearance, even though their physical condition has a bearing on their social status and survival. We only care about cravings and bingeing and eating all the 'wrong' foods because of its effect on our appearance. The fault lies at the door of your hormones which drive most of our desires. If you went mad yesterday and ate the entire tin of biscuits, you'd probably put it down to the time of the month, the stress of work, your post-baby blues, ovulation pain or bloating. Having said that, we have one advantage over the animal kingdom, it is called willpower. Without willpower and the ability to harness a positive frame of mind, our hormones would rule every aspect of our lives.

## Mental Attitude

Well, I'm glad I'm not an animal and I prefer the sophistica-
tion of humans, but we seem to have gone too far in our
pursuit of the perfect life. Stress can be caused by a lot of
things, by the unrealistic pressures you put on yourself, both
in your life and your looks for example, but as you'll learn
later when I talk about the roles of stress and adrenalin in
making you fat, it leads to a range of unhealthy responses
like over-eating, and we all know what that can result in.
Lots of overweight people are not remotely bothered by
their appearance, so it's not the weight itself that matters,
but what you think about it.

Some people thrive on stress, so a factor in overcoming
body chaos is your mental attitude. Having trouble sticking
with your diet? Lacking motivation or willpower? Or simply
unable to understand why you can't stick with it when
you're so well motivated? The section on mental chaos gives
some answers to those tricky mental gremlins which inter-
fere with your willpower and threaten to overwhelm you
with negative thoughts. So don't panic. Help is at hand!

When a new client comes to me, she feels totally alone.
She says that her body has taken over and she is simply
dreading whatever it is going to do next. She feels that life is
unfair, her friends all manage to look wonderful with only
half the effort she is putting in, and she has exhausted every
avenue to successful good looks. She can't shift that last
stone despite sticking to her diet to the letter, her thighs are
huge even though she goes to the gym six days a week, and
to cap it all she's bloated and tired out most of the time. If
she does have good days she spends them dreading the
inevitable bad ones ahead. My first job is to calm her, sort
out the mental from the physical chaos and embark on an
immediate plan of action with the right diet.

## What's Food Got To Do With It?

Your body is like a plant which wilts without water. It's like a dog sitting by the back door pining for a walk. Plants and dogs can't talk to you, but they let you know they're not happy. This is precisely what happens when you feel washed out or irritable: your body is wilting because it is working hard all the time and needs fuel. Think of it like a supermarket after closing time, when an army of shelf-fillers are busy re-stocking with produce. When you are relaxing or sleeping, your body is on overtime, re-stocking your supplies ready for the next bit of action. As well as replenishing your muscles with energy stores, your cells have to be renewed, your hair grows, bone is replaced, and old or worn-out tissue is being repaired or maintained. Your hormones are the regulators of this process, telling your body that it needs you to sleep, be alert or have another meal. As any diabetic will tell you, when the hormone insulin goes haywire and blood sugar falls too low, the resulting mental confusion is life-threatening. Food in the form of glucose restores the status quo for the diabetic. If oestrogen falls too low you can have hot flushes and low moods and although low oestrogen is undoubtedly something you'd want to see your doctor about, severe dieting and lack of food can render your fat stores so low that your oestrogen levels are compromised, and periods stop.

And it isn't just the quality of the food you eat that regulates your hormones. The time of day that you eat and the number of times you eat are also important. In the diet section I have given you several plans to choose from, using the foods that make the most difference to your hormone status. Whatever shape you're in now, you can turn your life around and be free from the pain of mood swings, anxiety, depression, weight gain and exhaustion.

With the exception of severe medical conditions which need medication and management, day-to-day fluctuations in hormones can be largely controlled by a combination of diet, exercise and your mental approach. The business of being you is an exhausting saga which only ends the day you die, and good nourishment is completely and utterly the most important factor in your life. Without it, you simply don't exist. Wake up to the body of your dreams with a clear head, lots of energy and optimism.

If you are currently suffering from raging hormones and body chaos, here's some reassurance before you start trying to change things:

- You are not alone. Body chaos is a common complaint so you are in the majority.
- You're normal. There's nothing wrong with you and you're not ill. Your body is doing what it is doing for a reason.
- Show your body who's boss. Take control of your body, learn how it works and don't collapse in misery because 'nothing's happening'. It's not a conspiracy.
- Don't panic. There are lots of ways to beat your problems so if something's not working, we'll find another way.
- Don't listen to scare stories like friends gaining three stone on HRT, caesareans ruining your muscles forever or how being a fat child means you'll always be fat.

Just concentrate on what's happening to you.

Body chaos is not about being physically or mentally unwell, and if you have serious physical symptoms you must see your doctor. But hormone fluctuations can have devastating effects, especially on your brain chemicals. In fact, these hormone adjustments are so marked that I think we women are heroic in managing to stay on top of it at all!

## Your Best Friend

The longest, closest relationship you will ever have with anyone is with yourself, so you might as well get along with yourself. Husbands leave, parents die, friends drift away and children grow up, but you stare in the mirror every morning and that same old person stares back at you. Hating yourself is like being permanently at war with your best friend. Knowing who you are is comforting. Being a brunette can be more than a straightforward colour choice, it can be your statement. I always say that I won't go grey – not out of vanity – for the same reason I won't go blonde. I'm a dark-haired person. I've always been dark, and my personality somehow goes with it. Suddenly being a fat person when you've always been slim, losing confidence to the point where you can't walk into a pub without shaking with fear when you used to be the local show-off – these are more than stages of life. The person you used to know has gone, and you miss her.

So in case you're feeling hopeless right now here are some facts:

- You can't stop yourself getting old but you can prevent ageing.
- If you want to be, you can be the same weight for the rest of your life.
- You can maintain as many youthful characteristics as you choose, such as a trim waist and toned legs.
- You can feel as lively as a young person for the next forty years.

## Here's What I'll Be Looking At In This Book

### Hormones
- The right balance?
- How it all starts – hormones and growth.

- How they control your moods.
- Hormones and weight – do I have to gain weight on the Pill or HRT?
- Why do I get this terrible headache?
- I can gain half a stone before my period – why?
- Why am I so depressed after my baby?
- How hormones protect you.
- The hormones of stress – how they hang on to your fat!

**Getting a fabulous shape forever**

- Starting young – exercise and body care for early teens.
- Can I have heavy bones? – what you really weigh, before you start.
- What, start exercise at my age?
- Why has all this fat gone to my stomach?
- Standing tall – perfect posture always turns heads.
- Too tired for exercise – how to cope when you're tired all the time.
- No time to work out – coping during exams or work.
- Weight training – the only way to stay ahead of the game.
- Exercise during and after pregnancy.
- How exercise protects you.

**Food chaos**

- Getting over the fear of food and weight.
- Stop weighing yourself all the time! – why it means nothing.
- What really happens to food when you eat it.
- 'I'm eating fat-free and I still can't lose weight!'
- 'I feel guilty when I eat' – getting over the fear of food.
- What you should eat when you're fifteen to nineteen.
- Fit but fragile? Nutrition for young athletes and dancers.
- Dieting to die for – why anorexia is a really bad idea.
- Bulimia at any age – what really happens inside you.
- Better nourishment during pregnancy.
- Getting your weight down after the baby.
- 'I can't be bothered counting calories' – why you should get a grip.
- Weight gain from thirty up. Does it have to be?
- 'It's all going round my middle!' – midlife crisis.

- 'But I'm not even menopausal!' – it's a shock but it always comes before you're ready.
- The final insult – 'retired from my job, not from life'. Weight management in midlife.

### Getting your mind round it all
- Getting to grips with gremlins – those nasty mental showdowns.
- Keeping up when you're down – anxiety and panic attacks – no need for pills – stress can make you fat – calm down for the sake of your figure.

## My Mission

My mission is simple: you are going to overcome your body chaos by starting from scratch. I have learned balance in my own life and I have taught others how to feel good, look good and stay slim for the rest of their lives. It is really so simple. Here is what you will do.

### Establish a Routine

Slim people always eat to a routine. That is why they are slim. They also seem to eat 'anything they want', which is also true. They eat what they want and they don't eat what they don't want, and when they've had enough, they stop. You might not think that you could ever master this technique, but you will. Fluctuations in your life occur at every level – your moods fluctuate, the ebb and flow of work – so achieving some order, balance and routine in your living habits is as sensible as having a car with good suspension – the road might be rough but you glide over the surface without noticing the bumps! Your body works to a routine. Your period comes every twenty-eight days and you sleep for seven or eight hours a night. Hormones follow a natural pattern: they wake you up, give you energy and alertness and make you sleepy. My mission is to help you to work with these patterns by establishing eating routines which complement them.

## Embrace Discipline

You will get some discipline into your life. Far from being a straitjacket, discipline will give you freedom. It may seem like a punishment to eat certain meals and reject others and to have to say 'no' to caffeine or alcohol or sweets, but far from this being the case, it is actually a punishment for your body to have them. By being disciplined you are going to stabilize your hormones and be free to enjoy life as you have never done before, and this is not an idle claim. With a small amount of discipline in the matter of exercise you can achieve many more enjoyable goals than you could before, simply because you will have energy and optimism. Discipline saves stress, it saves other people stress because they know where they are with you, and it cuts down on time and money by limiting your choices. Later in the book I will draw up a plan of action to point you in the right direction.

## Self-respect

This body is the only one you've got, and it has to see you through a lot of good and bad times. After all, if you treated a dog like you treat yourself and only took it out for exercise once a month, the RSPCA would soon be at your door! Many women hate themselves, show themselves little respect, and their hormones react with outpourings of adrenalin, missed periods and weight gain. I want you to learn more respect for your body, and realize that if *you* don't look after it, nobody else will. After all, you can't hand it over to someone to exercise, feed, wash and dress for you and hand it back with an invoice attached. Now wouldn't that be a good business to be in!

## Mental Chaos

I couldn't write a book about women's hormonal body chaos without touching on your mental attitude. Later in the book I talk about your perception of body chaos – being motivated to take control is one thing, having the willpower to stay in the driving seat in the face of opposition from friends, temptations and bad influences is quite another. It's not your fault you've got these chaotic hormones, but you need to take the lead, so later in this book I have a few suggestions for coping with that little gremlin in your head called willpower, who starts arguing with you every time you see a packet of chocolate digestives!

Read on and start the most important journey you have ever made – the road to overcoming your body chaos!

### Body Chaos – All in the Mind?

Body chaos is all in your mind. OK, you might argue that the headache you've had for the past few days linked with your savage demolition of the entire contents of your fridge and your limp hair are most definitely NOT in your mind, but let me explain. As women we suffer about forty years of relentless monthly pain and bleeding in varying degrees of severity for several days at a time, yet we more or less carry on as normal. If you were suddenly bleeding from anywhere else you'd cancel everything, stay home and call the doctor. You put up with periods because you have to. Mental attitude is one of your greatest weapons in overcoming body chaos. How you deal with your body's inconveniences depends on your perception of them. If you had a rope tied round your ankles and were ordered to jump off a bridge you'd be paralysed with fright, yet thousands do this every weekend when they make a bungee jump. The danger remains the same but the terror is removed, and while I cannot cure you of your anxiety or premenstrual syndrome, I hope I can help you to take them in your stride.

If something in your life isn't working, you must fix the right bit of it rather than take the scatter-gun approach and fire off blindly into the dark hoping you'll hit something. In my experience as a diet writer, somebody who hates her body will often paper over the cracks with the first thing she can think of, and this usually means that she embarks on a starvation diet. However, she probably doesn't hate her face or her legs and her real bugbear is her stomach, so cutting calories willy-nilly could actually be ruining the parts of her she likes, and this then reinforces her sense of failure. The fact is, you need a clear idea of what you want to achieve, and you should go about it in a structured way.

Another problem is rigid old habits. I can suggest that a main meal is taken at lunchtime and a lighter meal in the evening and even promise that this will make a difference, but time and again I'll be told that a small lunch and a hearty family dinner is what they're used to. I've no quarrel with that but, personally, if I were promised an end to my problems with this simple change, I'd at least give it a go. So be prepared for change and reassessment. After all, children and adolescents do it all the time. What do they say when you ask where their dolls are? What response do you get if you ask where the posters of their all-time favourite pop band are? The things they used to be mad about are all of a sudden babyish, boring and past it. Teenagers don't mind throwing all their ideas up in the air, discarding them and starting new ones without a backwards glance, yet adults seem stuck in their old routines. Routines are good, routines are vital for a happy life, but if your routine isn't working you've got to find a new one.

And what about that vast army of sickeningly lucky women out there? You know, the ones who sail through life able to eat whatever they like without gaining an ounce, and another lot who wouldn't know the depths of despair if it came and swallowed them up whole, right? Wrong.

Some women simply don't want the world to know that they aren't coping. Your friend might profess to not caring one jot about her body while she is secretly an aerobics addict. Your thin friend who amazes you with her diet of wall-to-wall chocolate might be bulimic. I've known all these sorts of people. But you must stop worrying about others. Just remember that you are unique and you have a unique body which requires unique care. If your friend is lucky to be slim while gorging herself on chocolate every night, let her get on with it.

## Mind Chaos

The mind can do funny things to you, and I should know. A pain in my leg and I'm worrying about how I'll get through next Christmas. Mind chaos is unique in the animal kingdom. Animals are spontaneous and instinctive and have no expectations, regrets or standards. They don't get embarrassed or make allowances for each other's off days, and my nine-year-old cat isn't fretting about how she'll cope when arthritis sets in and she can't climb trees any longer. By setting standards and benchmarks for ourselves we have the added dimension of either falling short of or exceeding our expectations. By far the most common reason for women's failure to maintain their figures and looks is the mental factor. Here are some examples of hormonal mind chaos taking over:

| Body Chaos | Mind Chaos |
|---|---|
| My weight is soaring and I don't know why. | I can't go out because of my body. |
| I exercise all the time but my legs are still unshapely. | My legs are so unshapely I hate them and keep them covered up. |
| My stomach feels fat and bloated. | My stomach's so big I won't let my boyfriend touch me and our sex life is nil. |
| I can't stop crying. | I'm so depressed I'm considering suicide. |
| I'm tired all the time. | I'm so tired I want to give up. |
| I can't stop bingeing. | I'll never get out of this binge-starve cycle, so why can't I be happy as I am? |
| I'm fatter than my friend. | It's not fair – my friend eats anything she likes and doesn't put on an ounce. |

It's incredibly easy to lose a sense of perspective, especially if you're reaching your teens or are isolated at home or in a job where you're left on your own a lot or travelling. One minute you simply hate your post-baby bump, the next minute you're panicking because you might be stuck with it for good. Your breasts might not be growing, but after a while you feel suicidal because they might never get any bigger.

## You and Your Food: Friend or Foe?

Many of my clients will tell me that they have a difficult relationship with food, when what they really have is a difficult relationship with their alter ego. One side of you wants to be this elegant, sophisticated woman in total control – in fact, being normal would be good enough – the other person inside your head sits at home stuffing food into her mouth. While you look at tempting trays of cakes and think 'no', she says, 'Oh, go on, one won't hurt.' You give in to her, and you hate her for her power over you. It's nothing to do with the food. Real food fanatics spend time choosing and preparing special menus, then they have dinner parties and invite other 'foodies' and the meal is discussed in minute detail and nobody overeats: they sample tiny portions; they enjoy the flavours. Most of all, they know when they've had enough and they pace themselves because tomorrow there'll be another lovely meal. With you, you're always promising yourself that you won't eat, so there becomes this terror that you'll never actually have another plate of chips or whatever. You feel that you're somehow missing out on this wedding buffet so you're jolly well going to enjoy every bit of it, and maybe have a bit extra while it's free. This dialogue with the other person in your head becomes a battle of wills, and it has nothing to do with the food. I remember talking once to a recovered anorexic who was glad she was well again, but bereft of the other person inside her head. 'Since I got well,' she said, 'I feel as if I've lost a friend.'

Hormones control many of your mental processes and, as you'll learn in the next section, food binges and chaotic eating will only upset your hormones even further. You are what you eat and your attitude is to do with what you eat.

Then there's good old willpower. I'm always frustrated that despite all the support I can offer someone, I can't actually have willpower for her. This is what I mean when I say that wealthy women have no advantages over the less well-off when it comes to dieting. People scoff and say you're crazy, what about all the gyms they can join, the personal trainers, the sheer time they can spend just working out and having fancy lunches? But I tell them that it's not like that at all: none of this gives you the willpower to succeed. If you really can't win the battle of the mental gremlins slugging it out in your head, you'll never lose weight, stick to a diet or doggedly stay for the full hour in the gym.

Later in the book, we tackle these issues head-on with what I hope is a light-hearted look at getting the better of those gremlins.

Chapter Two

# Hormones

Your hormones have a lot more to do with the person you are than you might believe. As women we tend to think about our sex hormones as the governors of our bodies and certainly much of the weight gain, bad moods, missed or irregular periods, bingeing and so on, which we call body chaos, are due to the hormones which control our reproductive system. But we also have a mass of other hormones which, together, regulate our lives to such an extent that one can only wonder at how we manage to stand up to the changes they inflict at all, rather than be surprised when we don't.

In the womb you are affected by your mother's hormones which come across from her placenta, so you are born with a dominance of maternal hormones which are gradually lost over the first few months of your life. Hormones are chemical messengers and they produce changes in certain cells. The word hormone actually means 'to urge on' which is precisely what they do, like a set of snooker balls which set each other off in a chain reaction. If one hormone fails it can have a disturbing effect on the others, with subsequent changes in weight, mood levels and so on.

Only tiny amounts of hormones are needed to produce powerful effects, and hormones are very precise. The first hormones which I am going to describe are those which are common to all of us, men and women. These are the hormones which regulate basic functions like our metabolic rate (the rate at which we use energy), sleep patterns and blood-sugar levels. We tend to be less well informed about them because we are probably not aware that any of these functions are due to hormones. If your energy levels are low, for example, and you have gained a lot of weight recently, do you need your thyroid testing or have you simply been having a lot of late nights and Chinese takeaways? Your uniquely female hormones, on the other hand, can fluctuate on an hour-by-hour basis, and you certainly know if your oestrogen levels have risen as they go about the business of preparing you for pregnancy. It is important to understand your hormones and it is also very interesting and might point you to areas of your own body chaos not addressed in this book.

## The Hormones Common To Us All

### Thyroid

The thyroid is a small, butterfly-shaped endocrine gland at the front of your neck weighing less than 28 grams, and the functioning of your entire body depends on it. Its job is to take up iodine from your bloodstream and synthesize two hormones, thyroxine ($T_4$) and tri-iodothyronine ($T_3$). The active hormone is $T_3$, which controls your metabolic rate, and $T_4$ is converted to $T_3$ by the action of an enzyme which is dependent on the mineral selenium. The thyroid sets the 'throttle' of your metabolism, so the more of these hormones you have the quicker your metabolism works; the less you have, the slower your metabolism. Your pituitary gland sends messages to the thyroid to produce these hormones and ensure that the right amount is made, and such is the importance of this system that it is responsible for the normal working of every organ, cell and tissue in your body. If this delicate system goes wrong, all your hormones can rage out of control.

People with an overactive thyroid feel stressed and exhausted but cannot get any rest. This condition is called thyrotoxicosis, and mostly affects elderly people. They feel hot, and overworked, and their functions become chaotic. There is wasting and weakness of the muscles, weight loss and a sense of being 'burnt out', but fortunately treatment for this condition is readily available.

An underactive thyroid is blamed by many women for unexplained weight gain and, indeed, thyroid problems are especially common in women, and are more likely to occur at the menopause or after childbirth. This makes diagnosis particularly difficult as it is often masked by the normal hormonal changes which take place at this time, with feelings of sluggishness, weight gain, joint pains and general puffiness being common symptoms of both conditions.

It used to be common to see people walking around with a goitre – a swelling in the neck caused by the thyroid gland enlarging to absorb any iodine it could find, which it needs to function properly, but a high-protein diet speeds up the activity of the thyroid by supplying the amino acid tyrosine from which thyroxine is produced. So to be sure of good thyroid function your diet should be rich in proteins, vitamin C and the B vitamins. Shellfish is rich in iodine, and kelp is a better source than table salt, which is usually iodized by the manufacturer.

There used to be a saying among doctors that the typical thyroid patient was 'fair, fat and forty'; the 'fat' because of the slower metabolism and forty, because that was the average age that thyroid problems presented themselves, but quite where they got 'fair' from, I'm not sure! Janine, forty-six, suffered from years of weight problems before she was eventually diagnosed:

I felt as if I was losing my mind. I'd had a good job as a division executive for a major high-street name, and had prided myself on my beautiful clothes, my size-ten figure and the way I was turned out generally. Put simply, getting fat was simply not an option for me; I suppose you could say that I was obsessed by my appearance. I carried on in that job until I was nearly forty then suddenly my husband Ian became very ill with multiple sclerosis and I gave up work straight away to look after him.

Life was different, but not so different that I stopped caring about myself. I'd go to the gym, take long walks and make sure that I ate a little less to make up for the hours I spent watching TV every evening, keeping Ian company. I can honestly say that I counted every calorie and made sure I got out for at least an hour every day, but I soon noticed that my clothes weren't fitting me any longer. This was bad enough in itself, but studying myself in the mirror a few weeks later, I saw noticeable hairs growing on my chin and upper lip where there'd been none before. I simply thought I hadn't been as vigilant as I usually was in spotting these things, so I dealt with them and made up my mind to be more careful in future.

Being so cold was my next nightmare, but I put this down to my increasingly inactive life. I soon noticed that I felt cold even after my aerobics class, a time when I had usually felt hot and sweaty. Catching sight of myself one day in a shop doorway, all I could see was a middle-aged, fat woman with dry, wiry hair and a look of coarseness about her. I panicked and went home to weigh myself, something I hadn't dared do for over a year. To my horror, I had gained nearly thirteen kilos since the day I left work.

I went to my doctor, but she was simply not interested. When she took my history she more or less closed the file and suggested that giving up my job and staying at home with Ian had simply made me eat more and become less active, which I suppose was true. I asked about the dry hair and the facial whiskers, but she just told me to go to a beauty salon for treatments. It's true I was starting the menopause and had noticed a few problems with that, but I couldn't agree with her. These young female doctors can be so dismissive!

I went through this hell for another year, but by this time I was feeling as bad as Ian, and he needed help more than I did. I then read a magazine article about an underactive thyroid, and it seemed to be talking about me. I saw another doctor and asked for a thyroid-function test, which came back showing that mine was slow. The doctor put me on a course of thyroxine.

If you expect your weight to suddenly drop and your old self come back immediately, it won't. It takes time, and I found being patient very difficult. But it DID work. Gradually I found my energy returning, which was half the battle, as it meant I could do more exercise. The weight slowly disappeared, and now I feel a lot more like my old self, about six kilos lighter, skin nice and soft again, and I've started some HRT tablets for the dwindling oestrogen so I've even got my sex drive back with a vengeance!

I'd say that you should never be put off by a bad GP, and don't be afraid of taking hormones or other tablets if they'll get you back to your old self. Thyroxine isn't some kind of miracle weight-loss pill though. If you have a bad diet and exercise habits, thyroxine will simply return you to your normal, flabby self, not endow you with a brilliant, size-ten figure! In future I am embracing exercise with a vengeance because I'm told it is the best thing for all your hormonal functions.

Recent research has revealed that up to one in ten women suffer from thyroid problems after having a baby, but on the other hand rushing to have your thyroid function tested needs to be done only after you have examined your eating habits and activity levels. Often as not, function is quite normal and it is simply your lifestyle which is the cause of those unwanted kilos.

## Adrenalin

Adrenalin – the so-called 'fight or flight' hormone, is secreted by the inner part of the adrenal gland, and it prepares your body for action by stimulating your muscles and circulation by providing instantly metabolized fat and carbohydrates as fuels. Adrenalin has a useful purpose: it keeps you alert, so that when there is a real threat it either arouses you to fight or recognize that the threat is too great and enables you to flee. Both **responses** need your body to be stimulated instantly and to operate at a high rate of efficiency, essential for people such as pilots and soldiers. It is the adrenalin which makes them able to do their job well, but too much adrenalin for too long can cause your body to become numbed and to shut down, leading to oblivious, dissociative states and panic disorders long after the event.

## Post-affair burn-out

Being exhilarated, in love and 'on a high' is a wonderful feeling. Some types of love affair thrive on the danger aspect: he might be married or you are leading a double life. Your meetings are intense and passionate, followed by periods of limbo, when you both wait to see each other once again. Normal life is about gentle ebbs and flows in daily activities, with intense excitement being replaced by other activities and duties which require attention, so to a great extent you forget the thrill you've just had because you have other things to do. When you are in a thrilling affair you have nothing when it stops. Periods apart are spent in a state of longing which is like a bereavement, and your body begins to crave the adrenalin high it now depends on.

Take the case of Suzanne, thirty-two, a lecturer in graphic design. Her life seemed humdrum but enjoyable, and she described herself as 'normal, boring and happy', until a couple of years ago when she met Andy, a soldier, who was about to get divorced but who was still living with his wife. The attraction was mutual and instant, and Suzanne fell completely and devastatingly in love with him. As Andy was based some distance away, their meetings only took place once a fortnight at first, then less frequently when he went away on exercises which were sometimes abroad.

However, the brevity of the meetings made them more intense, and Suzanne soon realized that theirs was a highly sexual, erotic affair, without many normal elements usually associated with two people in love. When he was away Andy would send flowers, letters and record audio cassette messages which spanned more than an hour of romantic ramblings. When they were together he would sometimes be moody and indifferent, sulky and introverted, then overwhelmingly affectionate.

Suzanne wanted to give him up but felt unable to do so, and there followed an intense year of high emotions and wild passion. Suzanne would sit by the telephone or race home from work to be there for a call or letter, often to be bitterly let down. Andy called all the shots and Suzanne witnessed herself becoming used and abused in a relationship she felt powerless to end. When asked why she carried on with Andy, she would cry and say she feared having nobody, then she would dry her tears and talk dreamily about the joy and excitement of being with her lover. The entire relationship was built on danger. Suzanne could not see that she was addicted, not to Andy, who was bordering on psychopathic, but to adrenalin. 'It's like going on one of those terrible fairground rides,' she confessed. 'You spend two hours in the queue for a two-minute, terrifying ordeal, but at the end of it you're so exhilarated you go straight to the back of the queue so you can do it again.'

The relationship eventually ended when Andy admitted to having had three other affairs at the same time as seeing Suzanne. Her tolerance and dependence collapsed and her health started to suffer. For the first time in her life she suffered panic attacks, then as they subsided she felt restless, exhausted, unable to concentrate and eventually severely depressed. She was prescribed anti-depressants, and although she is now much better, she does not feel confident enough to enter a new relationship.

These sorts of affairs are draining. Being in love in the normal way releases 'feel good' hormones which bathe your brain with calming chemicals which, while not masking the excitement of seeing your lover, don't indicate a state of danger. Adrenalin tells your body that it has to be ready for action, something from which even primitive man needed a break from time to time. Anybody who has been in this type of relationship will know that the stress is constant. You think about the person every waking moment, and that means your adrenalin is on permanent alert. In war it is known as being 'battle-weary', but it happens to us civilians too and the result can be depression, lowered immunity, weakness and either weight gain or weight loss.

## Adrenalin to save your life

More and more cases of allergy are hitting the headlines. You probably know about anaphylactic shock following peanut ingestion as one example. Interestingly, it is often reversed by administering adrenalin, so the reputation of adrenalin as a hormone simply associated with stress needs to be reassessed. It can frighten the life out of you, but it can also give you the courage to do something you would not normally do. For many people life would be boring without the odd adrenalin rush, and while there's no doubt that too much adrenalin can kill, given at the right moment, this hormone can literally save your life.

## Stress and weight gain

What do smoking, nail-biting, pencil-eating and chewing gum all have in common? Everything goes into the mouth! The second common feature is that you do them mostly when you are worried, pressured or simply working hard. You feel stressed, and for some reason you want to put something into your mouth. On some occasions you turn to food. So why does this happen?

The primitive mechanism which primes you for survival operates on a very basic level. Remember that adrenalin is there to enable you to have the strength to take life-saving action, and the minute you spring into action, marshalling the forces of your heart, lungs and powerful muscles, your energy stores are being raided. Calories get used like petrol in a Rolls Royce. The minute you stop for a rest your body needs to replenish its energy supplies in double-quick time in case you go into action again. You might be ready for a night slumped on the sofa watching television after a hard workout at the gym, but your body doesn't know this. It only knows that it has few energy stores left, so its response is to increase your appetite and you therefore want to eat. The hour or so immediately after vigorous exercise is the best time to eat because the calories will be used to replenish glucose supplies in your muscle – the ones which were so aggressively raided when you leapt into action, or on a more realistic level, had that punishing squash game or aerobics class. Your body's first concern is always to get you back into fighting condition as quickly as possible, rather like a racing car's pit-stop. Food eaten after exercise can still be turned to fat if there are more calories than you need, but eating after exercise is like the difference between putting cotton wool into a furnace, and holding a log over a candle. Both burn, but at vastly different rates!

As I explained earlier, stress provokes the same physical response, flooding your body with adrenalin. Your body only recognizes fear or alertness so it draws on your reserves to feed the tension. Naturally this means you start running low, and the eating response kicks in. You might chew pencils, bite your nails, light a cigarette or chew gum, but if you turn to food that is where the weight can become a problem. If you think about it, when tension subsides after a particularly worrying time, you head for food, sometimes eating in a frenzied fashion, without tasting or savouring it. The trouble is, you haven't been exercising so your muscles aren't exhausted or depleted of their stores. You've been ready for a fight which never took place, so the calories you eat are not needed for energy and are stored as fat. If you turn to cigarettes to relieve the tension, then of course you'll burn off a few calories and be one of those typical thin, nervy types. Stress can make you ill, it can make you thin and it can make you fat. Whatever else it is, it isn't good for you. So try the Anti-stress Diet on page 218.

So stress can cause heart attacks and other health problems because fat cells are mobilized but not used but there is a simple answer to this problem – if you feel stressed go for a walk. All you need do is use those fat cells in your muscles and burn off the energy, so get up, go downstairs or round the block or whatever. This is why they say that exercise relieves stress. The worst scenario we've all experienced is the one where you're held up in a traffic jam for hours, all hyped-up with no outlet for your mobilized fat stores and flight response. When you say you can feel stress 'coursing through your veins' in situations like that, it's a pretty accurate description.

## Adrenalin and panic attacks

Adrenalin isn't just released in times of stress, it is also triggered by low blood sugar and it can lead to panic attacks or make you feel generally weak and unwell. People who constantly over-stimulate their adrenalin by eating erratically are asking for trouble with their hormones, moods and weight.

Not being properly physically and mentally equipped and living in a chaotic body are like setting off for a European touring holiday in a beat-up car which has failed its MOT. It's like filling a racing car with diesel or feeding a champion racehorse a few leftovers. What you put in, you get out in performance. If you are permanently tired, stressed, under the weather or having rows with people, you are robbing yourself of your physical defences, and without these defences you are going into battle with half your ammunition. Many high-flyers scoff at this notion because up to now they have been lucky, but face it – however big a deal you're in the middle of, you can't work efficiently if you can't get a decent night's sleep and you can't get a decent night's sleep if you never get any fresh air or exercise.

## Growth Hormone

Night and day, your pituitary gland, situated at the base of the brain, is busy at work producing growth hormones. In children, it sends messages to the cells at the ends of the arm and leg bones telling them to divide, and as they do the bones get longer and the child grows. In the 1980s it was discovered that growth hormone was involved in more than just growth, and so had been misnamed. It was found that adults need it as much as children, though in smaller quantities. Growth hormone regulates the flow of sugar into muscle and fat, and helps the body to adapt to fasting if no food is available. With such a vital role it can be catastrophic if things go wrong. Growth hormone has a role in maintaining general well-being and so to the extent to which happiness and joy are derived from life. This has a major impact on success in the workplace and success in forming relationships.

A healthy pituitary gland needs a diet which is particularly rich in vitamin E.

## Melatonin

Melatonin is causing a great deal of excitement around the world. Discovered in 1958, melatonin is now a fashionable hormone, due in part to the claims that it is anti-ageing. Many experts disagree as to whether melatonin actually keeps the body young and the consensus is that there is no firm evidence.

Melatonin is made by the pineal gland, a tiny pea-sized hormone production centre which is crucial to our internal body clock and, as night falls, the gland awakens and begins its job releasing tiny quantities of melatonin. This triggers your body to prepare for sleep. As the sun rises the pineal gland senses the light change and the production of melatonin stops. The human body clock runs slightly longer than twenty-four hours, so each day that bit extra has to be re-set back to twenty-four hours. If our body clocks weren't re-set by melatonin we'd be twenty minutes out of synchronization every day, so production of melatonin is vital.

Melatonin makes you sleepy and lowers your body temperature, so it is a contributory factor in tiredness and poor performance in night workers. Jet lag is a result of your body clock being out of sync, and melatonin is now being taken by people who have to travel a lot across different time zones. Though we are never actually deficient in this hormone, blind people frequently suffer from an altered body clock because of their brain's inability to get enough melatonin released. In particular, blind people often suffer from poor sleeping patterns due to their erratic melatonin release, because daylight is registered through our eyes.

Increasingly, people are trying to take control of their hormones even when there are no medical indications that this is necessary, but taken at the wrong time you can seriously confuse your system. It is also not as simple as just taking a tablet. Taking hormones only works if you take precisely the right amount at the right time, and such is the concern over people popping pills without good reason that, in this country, over-the-counter sales of melatonin are now banned. Melatonin is a good example of the powerful effect hormones can have on our bodies. Advances in science now allow us to have some control over its production, but should we be interfering, especially when the timing and dose is crucial? We just don't know the long-term implications of manipulating this powerful hormone.

## Cortisol

Cortisol and adrenalin are two hormones that work hand in hand as they are both hormones of stress and alertness. Cortisol is produced by the cortex of the adrenal gland, and it is the slow rise of this hormone which causes melatonin to fall, waking you up and (hopefully) making you feel more energetic: it could almost be called the 'motivating hormone'. One reason why it is so hard to wake properly if you are disturbed in the middle of the night is that melatonin is still present and cortisol has not yet been stimulated. This hormone, which makes you feel alert and positive, is the reason why the early mornings are the best time to exercise.

When you are stressed, two hormones come into play – adrenalin and cortisol. The problem with cortisol is that it has an important effect on your immune system, and when cortisol is being overworked, your immune system becomes seriously compromised. Hence, people who are continually working under pressure are prone to more colds and viruses than their laid-back colleagues. So it pays to give yourself space from time to time, and not to be afraid of saying that you can't do something.

## Insulin

Insulin is secreted from the pancreas, a vital organ near your stomach, and regulates the amount of sugar in your blood, effectively monitoring each little tweak of the blood-sugar level like a spider sensing a movement on its web. Insulin and blood-sugar levels are something you'll be hearing a lot about as this book progresses, because insulin is an important hormone in weight management, and blood-sugar levels are the little devils behind a lot of the chaos you might be experiencing. Low blood sugar can make you depressed, tired or panicky, high levels can cause irritability.

Insulin influences the way you metabolize your food and causes high sugar levels to be stored as fat. Natural sugars are found in carbohydrates where they are bound up with a variety of other nutrients. This means that the body does not absorb the sugars too quickly because it has a considerable amount of digesting to do to break down the complex food to get at the sugar molecules, and so the sugars are released slowly over a period of time into the blood stream giving continuous energy. Refined sugar, on the other hand, is already broken down and so the glucose in it is rapidly absorbed making blood-sugar levels rise, and producing a fast insulin response. The excess sugar is stored as fat and you get a short, sharp burst of energy. This huge production of insulin can result in symptoms of hypoglycaemia such as light-headedness, shaking, fatigue and irritability.

Too much sugar in the blood is life-threatening, so an efficient insulin response is important and the choice of which carbohydrate foods to eat is important. Carbohydrates have what is called a 'glycaemic index'. This has been discovered by scientists in tests in which a volunteer is given a measured amount of carbohydrate. The blood is then tested every fifteen minutes after the carbohydrate has been eaten. A food with a high glycaemic index enters the blood quickly, forcing up sugar levels, then drops again within about an hour. You probably assume that this only applies to sweets and chocolate – the typical 'sugar kick' foods mistakenly used by people like office workers whenever they start to slump over their desks in mid-afternoon – but in fact potatoes, Cornflakes, white rice and root vegetables have a higher glycaemic index than choco-late. However, if you regularly suffer from mid-afternoon tiredness, a quick walk, a glass of water and an apple would do most for you. Food with a low glycaemic index enters the blood stream slowly and the effect lasts a couple of hours, releasing a steady stream of glucose to keep you feeling energetic and responsive even when you might be hungry for your next meal. Remember that hunger pangs indicate that your stomach is empty, not that your body has run out of fuel. The fuel has simply moved out of your stomach and onwards on its journey to do you some good, and if you couldn't eat for a while longer you wouldn't die. A more detailed list of everyday foods and their glycaemic index is given on pages 306.

In centuries gone by when diets relied heavily on unrefined foods such as whole grains, berries and fibrous fruits which have the type of carbohydrate which is released into the blood-stream slowly, insulin responses were also slower. Ancient diets were unrefined, cooking processes simple, and meals were consumed slowly, unlike the breakneck speed of eating in the street or the car which takes place nowadays. People laugh and say that eating on the run is unavoidable, but if they knew the effect on their pancreas they might think twice.

## Insulin and exercise

Exercise is vital for a good insulin response. This is going back to the spider in the web or the cat leaping into action when seconds ago it was soundly asleep. When insulin is sensitive it doesn't need much to produce the necessary effect, but a sluggish response is like trying to start a car which has been rusting in a garage for a year. That frustrating turning-over of the engine, the failure to respond, the over-use of the choke which results in the engine being flooded – in fact I can't think of a better analogy. Exercise improves insulin sensitivity, as well as providing a whole host of other benefits for your mind and body.

Being insulin resistant can be a major factor in weight problems because the carbohydrates you have eaten remain in your blood for longer. Increasing your physical activity and eating a low-fat and high complex carbohydrate diet will normally improve insulin resistance, and overweight or obese people can reduce their insulin resistance with a weight loss of about 10 per cent, so an individual weighing 95 kilos can reduce their weight by 10 kilos which will make a huge difference to their health.

Cardiovascular exercise is just another way of describing exercise which gets you sweating and breathless. Obviously there are guidelines which you should be given by a qualified professional who can meet and advise you personally, and you need medical approval before launching into a regime of gut-busting exercise if you have never done it before! Having said that, your body tends to be self-regulating, and the bottom line is that your heart and circulation need exercise as much as your arms and legs. Cardiovascular exercise helps prevent weight gain, so make it a regular fixture in your life.

The pancreas is the final blood-sugar regulator. When the mechanism is constantly over-stimulated by massive sugar surges from sweets, soft drinks and biscuits, the pancreas simply either becomes exhausted or so sensitized that it responds by producing too much insulin. This lowers your blood sugar to the point where you become hypoglycaemic

– resulting in listlessness and overwhelming muscle weakness. A good diet to keep insulin levels steady is one which balances high and low glycaemic-index foods, and provides a small meal every three hours. The Good Mood Diet is also very suitable for anyone suffering from regular low blood sugar.

## A Day In the Life of Your Hormones

### Daybreak

Your pineal gland senses the change in light, melatonin ceases production and cortisol levels rise, making you gradually more alert. Insulin levels are steady, but blood-sugar levels are low after the night's fast.

### 8.00 a.m. – breakfast

You eat your usual breakfast and blood-sugar levels rise (according to what you have eaten). If the food is high on the glycaemic index, such as Cornflakes, toast and marmalade, sweetened cereals, your sugar levels will rise quickly, insulin will rush out to redress the balance by forcing the levels down. If your breakfast is low on the glycaemic index, foods such as porridge or milky coffee, the insulin response will be slower.

### 9.00 a.m. – you arrive at work

You start work, and according to the type of work you do or the environment you have, your adrenalin levels rise. In particularly stressful situations, fat is released into your bloodstream, ready to marshal the forces of your muscles for combat. A fight does not happen, so the fat returns to your bloodstream, where it can now endanger your arteries.

### 11.00 a.m.

You begin to feel slightly tired and hungry as your blood-sugar levels start to fall again. You eat a biscuit, and insulin again rises slightly to redress the balance.

**1.00 p.m. – lunch**

Hungry, you go out for a large plate of pasta, garlic bread and a glass of wine and have ice cream for dessert.

**2.30 p.m.**

This sugar surge has triggered an enormous insulin rush. In mild cases you feel grim, overwhelmingly listless, and you crave something sugary, like chocolate. In many cases though, it triggers a more violent response and you suddenly begin to feel sweaty and you start trembling. Your heart is racing and you feel sick. Increased insulin production due to the large amount of sugar you have eaten at lunch reduces your blood-sugar levels, and your body now senses that you have too few glucose stores because you are in combat. Adrenalin is now pouring into your system, preparing you either to run from danger or stay and fight it out. Your racing heart is working to pump adrenalin and prepare your muscles for action, but it centres round your vital organs, leaving your extremities tingling as the blood supply is reduced. This is a panic attack.

**3.00 p.m.**

You have a biscuit and some sweet coffee which restores your blood-sugar levels.

**6.00 p.m.**

Your adrenalin rises again as you fight through the traffic on your way home and experience delays. Your body is preparing you for combat again as it senses stress, but you can only sit in your car, feeling tense. Fat is mobilized.

**7.30 p.m.**

You go to your aerobics class. Hard exercise releases 'feel good' chemicals into your brain which energize you. Your blood sugar is used up to feed your working muscles, so insulin is called upon once again.

**8.30 p.m.**

You go home and eat dinner. Your muscles are depleted of the sugar glycogen, so the blood sugar is needed to replenish stocks. You do not need as much insulin to drive levels down.

**10.30 p.m.**

Melatonin starts to be produced again by your pineal gland, as it senses the change in daylight. You begin to feel sleepy.

You go to sleep and the whole cycle starts again.

# Your Uniquely Female Hormones

## Becoming a Woman

When children are born, their sex hormones are not dominant, which is why little girls and boys see the opposite sex as a nuisance, and kissing an embarrassment! However, somewhere between the ages of eight and twelve things start to change. This change happens in the hypothalamus, a specialized part of your brain which houses many control centres like your day/night rhythms, your moods, your weight control and your cycle of periods or menstrual clock. The hypothalamus produces a very powerful hormone called gonadotrophin releasing hormone (GnRH) which is basically responsible for telling your pituitary gland to start off your periods. But something else has to happen first before this reaction is triggered – you have to weigh 50 kilos.

### What happens next?

There is a generator in your hypothalamus gland sending pulses of GnRH into your bloodstream. At first, this happens just a couple of times during the night, but then pulses start to occur during the day. Eventually the GnRH has the strength to 'fire' your pituitary gland which then releases the follicle stimulating hormone (FSH). Levels of FSH rise, and in return the hormone oestradiol is secreted which starts to prepare the lining of your womb. This doesn't mean your first period is about to start, but the wheels have been put in motion. These levels of hormone fluctuate quite a lot, but they have to become strong and once you have reached that level, your egg is released, and you have started a cycle of fertility which will continue, pregnancy and other problems permitting, for the next forty years. This, then is the beginning of our true body-chaos story, for it is the female sex hormones which cause the greatest havoc.

I am not a doctor, so problems with heavy periods, infertility or premature menopause are not dealt with in this book. These are conditions for which you must seek medical advice.

## Adolescence

Adolescence can be stressful. One minute your parents are demanding that you do as they tell you, the next they are asking you to make major decisions, like what you are going to do for a living! Your body is changing before your very eyes, and all the while you're being expected to pass exams and apply for jobs or university places. Adolescence is about competition. You're competing for your place on the ladder, your place in life's line-up and of course you are competing for the biggest prize of all – a mate. Like it or not, nature is preparing you for motherhood. You might not want children, might hate the sight of men and have the nesting instinct of a felt-tipped pen, but your hormones aren't put off. Your choices are valid and modern life is reflecting these choices but your body is primitive. We talk of inner turmoil and ticking body clocks but nature doesn't work like this. If you really want a battle on your hands, you'll never get a better one than the struggle between you and Mother Nature.

So right now you're discovering who you are and it's time to experiment. Do you really want to stick with dark hair? Is short hair your style or will you set your own trend and go curly? Finding an image that feels comfortable is quite normal – celebrities and pop stars pay advisers thousands of pounds to come up with a 'look' and a branding for them – so experiment! Once you get a look you're comfortable with, you've made an important first step. Then you must learn how to look after the new you, so you have a body which gives you years of trouble-free service.

If you're into competitive sport or are simply a keen dancer who might be making it her career, you'll be at the peak of your excellence right now. Being lightweight is a major component of perfection, but there are a great number of factors apart from weight which are involved in success – ability, mental preparation, good training, fitness and strength, for example. There has to be a keen dedication and commitment to perfection and excellence, and unfortunately although this is admired and respected, it can often endanger future health.

## Your cycle

Now your cycle is up and running with any luck you can weather the ebbs and flows without too much disruption to your life. I have found that most of us can bear the normal fluctuations because – well – we have to! But when you feel that the cycle has somehow got out of control – that it has ceased to be normal or predictable like the usual monthly event – then you get distressed. All women have parts of the month when they feel absolutely fabulous in one way or another and other parts of the month when they feel terrible, and it's easy to let the bad times take over. To calm matters a little, let's look at what happens during the stages of your normal menstrual cycle.

## Oestrogen

Oestrogen is the hormone which controls the first two weeks of your cycle, until your egg is released from your ovary.

Oestrogen is an important hormone which has a particular effect on your moods. Considering that the right balance is not always struck, it's not surprising that so many of us have such sudden and upsetting mood variations. High oestrogen can make you anxious and irritable, low oestrogen can cause depressions. Some very high levels of oestrogen are also thought to be responsible for headaches. These were a often a side-effect of taking the old-style, high oestrogen level contraceptive pill of years ago.

## Progesterone

Progesterone's job is to prepare the lining of your womb for a fertilized egg. It has a calming and slightly sedative effect, and when it reaches its peak around mid-cycle you can find yourself feeling washed-out, tired and woolly-headed.

All being well, your normal hormonal cycle runs for between 21–35 days, usually 28 days. Considering that on almost any given day of the month something is happening to either prepare you for a period, make you have a period or get you back to normal after your period, I think it is amazing that we know how we genuinely feel at any one time! Here's how it all works.

If you look at the chart opposite, you will see that in the first half of your monthly cycle your hormones are governed by oestrogen, while progesterone is in control from mid-cycle onwards. It is the progesterone which takes over when conception has occurred, closing down your cervix and holding everything in place to protect the embryo. Progesterone in the right doses has a calming effect, but when progesterone is particularly low it is thought that it causes PMS.

## A month in the life of your reproductive hormones

### Day 1

Your period starts. The pituitary gland activates FSH which starts the process of maturing a new egg in one of your ovaries.

### Days 3–7

Your period is over. The new ovum starts moving to the surface of your ovary. A follicle starts producing oestrogen. This makes the lining of your womb thicker, in readiness for the fertilized egg to have a place to settle.

### Days 12–16

Ovulation happens around this time, mid-cycle. Your body makes luteinizing hormone (LH) to help the mature egg to burst through the ovary. The hormone progesterone prepares the lining of your womb further, and if the egg is fertilized it lodges in the lining. You start to feel

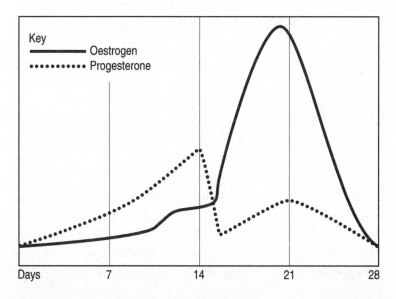

Key
———— Oestrogen
•••••••••• Progesterone

Days    7              14              21              28

hungrier, and the high progesterone level makes you lack energy. PMS may start.

**Day 20 onwards**

The egg travels down your fallopian tube to your womb. Oestrogen and progesterone levels fall. The egg and the thick womb lining are not needed so they disintegrate and travel down to be washed out, and this is your next period. Higher testosterone levels mean you might be more aware of the opposite sex and feel sexier, but you might also be more aggressive, hence the rages of pre-menstrual tension.

So you have this continuing cycle whose only purpose is pregnancy. Hormones are poured in to thicken the lining of your womb ready for a fertilized egg to settle in and together with the hormone progesterone, which comes into play at mid-cycle, they are believed to be responsible for the feelings of tightness, bloatedness, not being able to hold your tummy in and irritability. However, drops in blood sugar are the most usual causes of sudden outbursts of irritability, more of which later in the chapter Hormone Hell. As most of us know, the symptoms go when the lining is shed at your period.

## Not quite hitting the right note

In your teens, these pulses of hormones have yet to get established into a cycle, which is why you might get different lengths of time between bleeds. Anything from two to six weeks is normal, and even if you miss periods completely it isn't necessarily a cause to see your doctor if you feel well otherwise. Reasons for periods stopping can be linked to emotional distress and low body weight, although in adolescents it is also likely to be a 'blip' in the establishing of your cycle. Periods also cease in young women who are into competitive sport or dancing, and who might have a very low percentage of body fat, but there is a sensible reason for this: a woman must always be able to sustain a pregnancy because nature's imperative is for the species to survive. This is why we all feel we carry rather too much fat in our abdominal, hip and thigh regions, ready to be called upon in a crisis. If you have very little body fat nature decides that it's sensible if you don't conceive, so you stop ovulating and you don't get a period. Clever, isn't it?

The greatest hormonal effect at this time is on your emotions. If you find yourself swinging from one emotional extreme to the other it's likely to be because of frustration and continual battling. Battling with friends, boyfriends, authority figures, your parents and yourself. People cry because of tension, rather than sadness, and being in love can be a monumental frustration. In some ways of course, teenagers have it made when it comes to love because they have more choice than any other sector of society, but the downside of there being hundreds of boys on the market is that there are also hundreds of girls out there too. If there was ever a time to be sure your hair looked good and your thighs slim, it's now, but be careful. If you start a diet by simply not eating for hours on end, you will confuse your hormones even more as they need good nutrition to work properly. Later on I'll be giving you a desirable teenage eating plan, but it's important that you choose high-energy, high-nutrient food at this time, as you are now laying down the foundations for the next fifty years of your life.

## Having a Baby – and Afterwards

### Hormone changes in pregnancy

The next major incident in your body will probably be pregnancy, and when you know what happens to your body during pregnancy, it's amazing that you're ever the same again. Within hours of your egg being fertilized, the hormones are affected. Where the level of the hormones oestrogen and progesterone would normally start dropping after mid-cycle, in this case they continue to rise, and different hormones are produced. The level continues rising for several weeks, causing the characteristic morning sickness.

During the first few weeks that you are pregnant, more and more progesterone is produced, rising to fifty times the level it would normally be at its usual peak on Day 21 of your cycle. Another hormone, prolactin, is produced to prepare your breasts for feeding the baby, and amounts of hormones produced by your adrenal glands also double, changing your day/night rhythms, which might make you feel more active at night. Changes take place in all organs of your body, with production of oestrogen and progesterone now coming from the placenta rather than from your ovaries which leads to the dramatic fall in these hormone levels when your baby is born, when the placenta comes away with the baby.

## The chaos of pregnancy

While it's generally thought of as being a joyous time, having a baby is not exactly a piece of cake for most of us. If you've been the sort of girl who prides herself on her looks, the most stressful part of pregnancy is seeing the needle on the scales rise relentlessly. Then there's the aches and pains, the heartburn, the wanting to go to the loo every five minutes, the breast tenderness and the morning sickness. The good news is that it gets better the further into your pregnancy you go, although much depends on whether this is a first or a subsequent baby – in which case you'll be an old hand by now.

It goes without saying that it is vital to eat well during pregnancy, but many women still believe in the old adage of 'eating for two'. Well, in terms of calories and quantities you're not eating for two people, but you are eating for the *needs* of two separate people. And not just eating. Getting stressed, overdoing exercise, smoking, drinking alcohol and eating low-nutrient food are all going to affect that little person inside you, so show some consideration. Stop the cigarettes, stop the drinking and get the right nutrients. After all, the baby isn't the only one to suffer. Nature has seen to it that the baby's needs will always come first by ensuring it takes what it needs from its mother, so a bad diet will reflect badly on you. Body chaos is unfortunately the name of the game when it comes to late pregnancy, but what you really want to avoid is chaos afterwards.

## Like pulling out a plug

The fall in hormone levels after the birth is dramatic. For nine months you have had this high level of progesterone in your blood – fifty times higher than oestrogen and fifty to a hundred times higher than when you are not pregnant – and within hours of delivery the level has dropped to tiny levels. It is almost impossible for you not to register this massive decrease, but circumstances dictate that you are otherwise occupied. Visitors, the demands of the baby and a change in routine mean that you could well escape the 'baby blues' in a haze of euphoria – or exhaustion.

## Problems with coping

Lethargy and tearfulness are features of the first few weeks after childbirth, especially if you also have older children. Endless people looking into the pram or crib means less attention paid to you, which after nine months of people fussing around after you, making sure that you are comfortable and thriving, comes as a bit of an insult I always think. Your lustrous hair and smooth skin begin to show the typical post-pregnancy loss of sheen and condition, all of which add to the general misery, and I hardly need mention your shape. Sometimes the quick turn-around of hormones means there is not enough stimulus for the thyroid-stimulating hormone to be produced, which tells your thyroid gland to start releasing thyroxine. As discussed earlier, the thyroid gland controls your metabolic rate, and major body changes like pregnancy are common causes of thyroid disturbance. The symptoms of low thyroxine are lethargy, exhaustion, lank hair, which may fall out, chilliness and a slow pulse, but fortunately a simple test will tell your doctor if you need medication.

I always make it a rule when I see a new mother to ask after her and concentrate my entire conversation on her, without reference to the baby until the very end. She will want to be congratulated on producing such a beautiful/healthy/bouncing/unusual baby, but it seems unfair to base the entire conversation around it. Try to talk about other things she's involved with, how the local charity group misses her, how the office isn't the same without her and if she's a colleague don't forget to save up some office gossip for her, or ask her advice on a problem. If she has other children, talk about them too. The baby's important, but many new mothers feel as if they've been sidelined. *Be sensitive.*

## Endless exhaustion

Anaemia is another very common cause of exhaustion and crying fits, caused by blood loss at birth or a diet which simply has not been enough for the demands of the growing baby plus your own. Low potassium also leads to excessive exhaustion, especially if you have been taking diuretic tablets for swollen ankles or high blood pressure, because potassium is lost through natural excretion. Both these problems are best remedied through diet rather than tablets. There are several good diet ideas in the diet section, see page 239.

## Looking on the bright side

There are endless books and articles about depression, irritability and psychosis after having a baby, and severe symptoms should be referred to your GP or health visitor immediately. I suffered from bad post-natal depression after my first son was born, but it was a nightmare from which I recovered on my own, particularly when I stopped breast-feeding. Don't listen to scare stories. If you really want to make yourself miserable there are countless tales of woe, but many women don't just recover their figures and their mental equilibrium, they look better than they did before they were pregnant.

Hormones can run riot after having a baby and knowing what I do now I think I took the wrong course of action. I kept charts and diaries of my moods, and began to expect the worst when the appropriate dates came up on the calendar. 'Twenty-second of the month? Day 16 of my cycle? According to my chart I usually start to feel really bad around this time!' In short, you get obsessed with every heartbeat, every 'down' day and twinge. Remember that having a baby is a normal, natural occurrence for your body. Being tired is natural. Having a bit of extra weight, or having a few sloppy muscles is also quite normal, but it's not terminal. Obviously the best way to avoid having to diet again is to not gain the weight in the first place but, hell, being pregnant doesn't happen every day and it's understandable that you want to relax and feed yourself. But now the time's come to get back in shape, this time for good so step up the exercise and watch those forgotten calories.

## Mid-life – The Biggest Chaos of All

Articles about middle age used to feature silver-haired, laughing couples in cardigans, happily extolling the virtues of pension plans and golfing complexes in the Algarve. It was about freedom from care, empty nests and hiding those 'iffy bits' in the middle with flattering dress lines. Over-fifties' investment opportunities advertised on the television even today, suggest middle age as a time of gardening, grandchildren and the odd gentle game of bowls. How can they get it so wrong? Anybody in their early fifties right now was in their early twenties at the beginning of the 1970s when it wasn't so much a case of twinsets and pearls as platforms and flares, flower power and free love. You don't go through all that and suddenly crumble. These days, with more and more women having their first or subsequent children in their late thirties and forties the menopausal years are just as likely to be fraught with ten-year-olds and their homework, school runs and financial headaches. On the other hand, many women who did have their children early in life are enjoying their money and freedom at a time when they are fitter and healthier than ever before. It seems even more unfair then that nature decides to wind down your hormones just at a time when you need all the help you can get, and most women from the age of thirty-nine or so are suffering from some sort of hormone disruption.

The average age for the menopause is fifty-one, so if you're currently in your thirties or early forties, you might be thinking that you've got a while before you have to confront it. The menopause is something which happens to your mother, not you. Being menopausal has become a term of abuse. I heard a national newspaper columnist recently deliver this insult to an editor who got the better of him in a verbal tiff. 'Are you always like this, or is it only since you started your menopause?' he asked. I suppose this was meant to convey that she was old, dried-out and past it, rather than the sharp, authoritative, mature and attractive woman she really was, but it made me think. Why do people think they can be so offensive? You wouldn't say, 'Is it only since you got cancer?' or, 'Have you only been like this since you heard you were HIV positive?'

Being menopausal, of course, does *not* mean you're past it, although the word actually denotes the end of your periods and the end of fertility. You are truly at the menopause when you have had no periods for two years. So if that's the end of everything, when on earth is the beginning?

It's around the age of thirty-five. Scientists have long recognized that fertility gradually declines around the mid-thirties and the number of egg-containing follicles decreases. Levels of oestrogen start to fall off while the levels of FSH and LH soar. If you were about to dash to the doctor to complain that your hormones are out of balance, they are. Your GP will probably offer hormone replacement therapy, but hold on, the fluctuations in your hormone levels probably won't be consistent for some time yet, and what many women find at the very beginning of the peri-menopause – for this is what it's called – is that they have a bad month, then go back to normal service for the next six months or so – sometimes more than a year.

To illustrate this, here's Samantha's story. She's forty-six, a single parent of a ten-year-old and she works full time as a legal executive:

> I was thirty-eight at the time, and it had become a joke in my house that I would feel very hot at about 10.30 every evening, and come over all sweaty,

but I thought nothing of it because I had usually been to the gym earlier and I assumed it was my good circulation. About six months later I suddenly found that I was unbearably hot and sweaty at night, and my sleep was almost non-existent. On top of feeling hot, every time I tried to fall asleep I would feel as if I'd had a sudden fright and I'd sit up in bed feeling irritable and nervy. It didn't worry me, but it got me down because after a week I was desperately tired and I had a huge amount of work to get through at the office. I assumed I had some sort of virus, but then the depressions started. One night I came home from the gym and suddenly felt my mood plummet. It seemed to have nothing to do with how I was actually feeling – I mean my life's OK, I'm happy and everything – but I sat on my bedroom floor and bawled my eyes out for half an hour. I didn't feel I could confide in anyone because I'm in the sort of job where you'd do anything rather than admit that you're down.

Eventually I went to see my doctor because I couldn't see an end to this nightmare. She took a blood test and a week later I went back for the result. To my amazement and horror she told me that the test indicated that my LH was extremely high, indicating the peri-menopause, then she started writing out a prescription for HRT patches. I couldn't take it in. 'Am I having an early menopause then?' I spluttered through my tears. 'Oh no,' she replied. 'You're in the peri-menopause – the years leading up to the menopause. It's quite natural for your hormones to start getting ready for this event, but if you take HRT your oestrogen levels will go back to normal.' I noticed that she'd also prescribed some pills to take with the patches, which she told me were for the week prior to my period. 'You'll probably feel a little bloated and scratchy or tense,' she said, 'but that's just like any normal month of PMT. Your hot flushes and night sweats will vanish, and that's the important thing.'

I took the prescription, got my patches and pills then sat at home looking at them. You see, I'd never suffered from PMT in my life before, so being told that I'd have thirteen rotten, irritable weeks every year seemed a poor exchange for curing my hot flushes. I decided to give it another fortnight, and if I still couldn't sleep, I'd start using them.

Needless to say, my flushes stopped the following week. I didn't have any more for nine months and I felt good. I missed one period that year, the following year I missed three and it wasn't until early this year that the hot flushes started again with a vengeance and I haven't had a period for months.

All together I've swapped thirteen weeks of tension for a few days of moodiness, which I think is a good exchange.

I went for a consultation with a private endocrinologist just so I could understand everything. He told me that the symptoms of the peri-menopause were worse at the beginning because the hormones were fluctuating so dramatically, and that as the years went by they'd probably get better as my hormones dropped to insignificant levels. I never get any mood swings now, I feel energetic still because my job is very interesting and I have a good social life, and all I did have were the flushes which I have to admit were pretty draining, but they've now stopped. I found the disturbed sleep too much to take, but overall I'm glad I didn't go straight onto hormone replacement too soon.

When I think that the GP just handed out that prescription it makes me mad. I just wasn't ready for it, but I can see that the doctor simply wants to make you feel better as quickly as possible. I'm only forty-six now, and I've been told that a good diet and plenty of exercise can help me cope with my chaotic hormones. This diet includes things that soothe and calm, such as milk, cheese and chicken, and excludes things like caffeine, too much alcohol and sugar, which would make me even more irritable than I am already. Actually, I've always liked a nightly drink and thought that nothing would ever stop me having my 'tincture', but now the whole idea of getting slightly flushed with alcohol on top of night sweats well, it's such an effective deterrent that I view alcohol as poison these days! I'm also an advocate of exercise. I don't know if knocking myself out at aerobics is simply a way of dulling the pain, but I don't actually care. I've lost weight and regained my waistline, and it channels my aggression! I honestly don't think there's any substitute for good old natural oestrogen, so if anyone out there is thinking she can take a few evening primrose oil capsules and wave goodbye to the menopause, I'd say think again. The name of the game is finding a way of coping. It's not so bad!

I would agree with Samantha. Somebody said to me recently, 'But you make it sound so dreadful!' and I thought, 'Are you crazy?' Some people have fewer problems than others, that's true, and other people are simply glad to be free of the monthly curse, but on the whole I'd be hard pressed to find anything good to say about the menopause.

Samantha's story is typical. Nobody tells you that the change of life starts as early as it does. How you react to these changes is a personal thing, but it's usually the mental rather than the physical symptoms which cause the greatest distress. Most women have spent a tough few years getting their career in order, building up their resources and having a family, and it's now that they feel they have the money, time and energy to go out and have a good time. To have Mother Nature suddenly announce that you're infertile and ageing is a shock. The change is non-reversible. You can keep your figure and have the complexion of a teenager, but you can't dictate terms to your hormones. What I can promise you though, is that you can keep your lovely figure, not gain weight and feel bright and youthful again, and have a better future than you thought possible.

## How does all this happen?

When you are young and your cycles are established you pump out measured, rhythmic doses of hormones which stimulate your pituitary gland to secrete two other hormones. So far so good. By the time you reach thirty-five the amount of follicles has fallen, and the ones left behind die off more rapidly. Once the number of follicles drops below a certain level the fine tuning of hormones that you have taken for granted starts to go a bit haywire and this loss becomes self-perpetuating. The curtain finally falls around the age of fifty-one, when production of hormones ceases totally and your periods stop.

It is not the hormone levels themselves which cause body chaos, but the wild fluctuations. The pulses of hormones in young women need no extra help (although they do quite frequently go haywire) but as time goes by they get more erratic. I am reminded of those fairground games where you test your strength by hitting an anvil with a hammer in order to make the bell at the top of the column ring. More often than not the anvil isn't hit hard enough and the bell doesn't ring. In a normal cycle your level of oestrogen rises, this triggers FSH and the process releases an egg which travels down to your uterus. In the peri-menopausal period, fluctuations from the normal pattern have started because your oestrogen levels are lower, consequently you have trouble triggering FSH, and levels get higher and higher like the fairground anvil and bell game. The feelings you get can be either nothing at all or headaches or hot flushes, and there's a variety of other symptoms which might or might not be connected to your hormones.

Always bear in mind that there are social and lifestyle factors influencing your body, such as your impossible mother-in-law, overbearing boss, or the fact that your over-time money hasn't come through. These stresses cause considerable physical upheaval so don't underestimate them, but do go and ask your doctor for a blood test. Depending on the health budgets they might give you one, or you can pay for one to be done privately. None of this will alter the unpalatable facts, but at least you'll be armed with some knowledge which you can act upon.

The timing of the menopause is dictated by your brain. For many years scientists believed that it was the ageing ovaries which caused the increased loss of follicles, but it is now thought more likely that it is your ageing brain. In young women the pituitary gland pumps out LH in steady rhythmic pulses, but when you reach your late thirties, even if your cycles are normal and you are having regular periods, the release of LH becomes erratic. The pulses are longer but less frequent, and if you are peri-menopausal you will have high levels of FSH in the first week or so after your period. This happens because your hypothalamus is sending out low signals of GnRH, and it is responsible for those notorious hot flushes.

## Hot flushes, night sweats and panic attacks

Samantha has already described her experience with night sweats and hot flushes, but of course everybody's experience is different. I happen to believe that many panic attacks are in fact triggered by hot flushes, and panic attacks tend to feed on themselves. As you feel worse you worry about what is happening to you so the panic continues, especially if you are in a confined space or feel trapped by circumstances. Seeing that your hormone status is always a finely balanced affair, it seems likely that a slight shift, a slightly irregular 'pulse' of hormones which I have already explained – can easily trigger a flush which you won't have been expecting. So what does a hot flush feel like?

Many women experience a slight warning, a feeling in the chest that something dreadful is going to happen, like remembering that you've left an egg boiling when you're halfway to the airport. From there the flush spreads upwards to your neck and face. They can be very powerful or only slight, they can last a few minutes or a few seconds. Many women report flushes so bad that they have to sleep apart from their partners and never get a good night's rest. They feel as though they are dripping with sweat all over, even down their legs. After the flush, you can feel uncomfortably clammy and cold, and so it goes on.

It is not known exactly what causes hot flushes, but it is thought that it is not the actual level of oestrogen which matters, but the fact that it is falling. The fall disturbs the hypothalamus in the brain which upsets the centres which control heat in your body.

## At long last – freedom!!

The menopause itself is said to be complete when you have had no periods for two years. This is said to be the most satisfying time for many women. Rather than describe it myself, I'll leave it to Ruth, who is fifty-eight.

I had a lot of problems with mid-life. To be honest, I was a very pretty young woman with plenty of boyfriends, good jobs and no money worries. I had my four children young, and I can't pretend they weren't a handful, but we got by somehow. I rather lost my twenties to motherhood and being a housewife, then in my thirties I had more freedom, I retrained as a beauty therapist and opened my own salon. Life seemed completely perfect, I'd also divorced and was back on the market aged forty-one. I can't tell you what a fabulous time I proceeded to have for the next few years, that is until I felt the change kicking in, and then it became misery.

I didn't have a bad time because I took HRT from the word go. I didn't gain weight and I kept myself looking good, but inside my head I just lost it. People would look at my date of birth, or find out that my daughter was pregnant and therefore work out that I was nearly a grandmother and they treated me as if I was past it. Coming up to fifty was a nightmare because in my head I was thirty. Missing maybe four or five periods at a time seemed to reinforce this middle-age thing, and I nearly went off my head. You see, I was too near to youth to let it go. I looked in the mirror and saw what I'd always seen, I could do everything as I'd always done it – yet I felt overlooked and ignored.

My periods stopped completely four years ago. I then remember having a conversation with someone about chocolate cravings and those terrible rages you get before your periods and I thought, 'Oh, I'd forgotten about them.' I hadn't wanted to eat the fridge bare for years, and I no longer got moody or irritable. I was sitting in church one Sunday and I suddenly looked round at the dozens of women there, and I thought, 'At least two-thirds of you are probably having really rotten periods right now – or getting ready to have them or worrying about being pregnant – or not pregnant!' – and I felt this wonderful rush of relief. It wasn't awful being an older woman after all. I'd spent all this time feeling sorry for myself, and all the time people were asking my advice about things and I could really trade on all my experience. At the salon, I'm the only person who can boast thirty years in the business, which gets me a lot of respect. My hormones are pretty well dormant now, and the only way I can describe the effect is 'serene'. When you're young, you have 'times of the month' all the time – your body is either getting over a period, getting ready for one or somewhere in the middle, and you hardly have two days when you feel great. Post-menopausally, it feels like the landscape has been ironed out flat. There's no moods, no looking at calendars, no pains or bloating – in fact, I love it. Why older women think they're on the scrapheap I can't imagine. We're the seniors, the masters!

This then is the end of the hormone story – of your female sex hormones that is, because of course your other hormones, your insulin, thyroid and so on, carry on working until the day you die. Indeed, assuming that you die of natural causes, it is a hormone action that will determine your death.

But what about the chaos? I have already said that many women sail through life without a moment's chaos, but maybe they are just so busy they don't notice, perhaps they are stoical or possibly they have just forgotten! Whatever the case, we've all known what hormone hell means, but here are a few reminders or warnings about what might be lying ahead for you!

## Hormone Hell

There's nothing quite like the hell of hormones but what you eat and how you eat can really relieve the symptoms. Men can be understanding, but there's no way they could ever really understand. This section is one which I can con fidently promise I am writing from personal experience!

## What are Premenstrual Tension and Premenstrual Syndrome?

*'For half of the month I feel good, and the other half I'm like an axe-murderer with PMT. My life is hell – is there anything I can do other than go on the Pill?'*

PMT refers to the irritability and tearfulness that we suffer, whereas PMS or 'premenstrual syndrome' describes a whole host of symptoms including backache, leg ache, headache, nausea, depression and tearfulness, food cravings, anxiety, palpitations, sweats, itchy skin, sleep disturbances and so on. If you look at the chart on page 47, you'll see that oestrogen controls the first half of your cycle until the egg leaves your ovary, then progesterone is in control from mid-cycle onwards, and it is progesterone which takes over when conception has taken place, closing down the cervix and holding everything in place to protect the growing embryo. In the right dose progesterone has a calming effect, but when it is particularly low it is thought that this is the cause of the anxiety, irritability and other symptoms of PMS.

## Outbursts of Rage

This happens when your blood-sugar level has gone too low, especially among non-breakfast eaters, your body reacts to correct this imbalance by pushing out adrenalin which releases extra sugar to help raise your blood-sugar levels. As you learned earlier on, adrenalin is the hormone of 'fight or flight', and when adrenalin is suddenly released in a rush like this it can cause a feeling of fury and fight-fever. This stressed sensation results in a craving for sugary foods to help restore the balance, and this in turn leads to high blood-sugar levels. To correct these, insulin is released to force your blood-sugar down again to an acceptable level, which can leave you feeling tired, listless and tearful. The common end result of this depressing vicious circle is weight gain, unwillingness to exercise because you feel fat and further feelings of lack of self-worth.

## I Just Crave Food All the Time!

There are cravings and there is the plain hunger that comes with hormone hell and body chaos. When you crave food it is generally one type of food and chocolate, cheese, biscuits or ice cream come high on the list. Quite why these foods are the most popular nobody really knows. It is thought that some of the properties of chocolate and cheese, for example, encourage the production of certain brain chemicals that are linked to sexual arousal and they are craved for this reason. Personally, I'm sceptical, but I'll leave the issue for another time. I happen to feel that these foods are simply available, without any kind of preparation, and they undoubtedly taste good. I often crave a jacket potato, but by the time I've microwaved it and then crisped it up in the oven, the feeling's worn off. Eating lots and lots of food for the sheer hell of it, or because you can't stop yourself, is another thing, but what makes you so hungry?

A desire to eat is not the same thing as being hungry. Strictly speaking, it's not possible to be hungry within about two hours of a normal meal, longer if you've had a heavy meal. It takes that length of time for food to be broken down and digested in your stomach, and this is the reason that you're advised not to exercise within two hours of a meal. Food then moves on its journey to the small intestine and this is when your stomach begins to register those tell-tale emptiness pangs.

Bingeing affects your hormones because of the things you tend to binge on – nobody binges on tomatoes or kippers, or if they do I've never heard of it – and this turns into a cycle of despair. Refined carbohydrates cause an insulin surge which later leads to low blood-sugar levels, and as you now know, these low levels make you want to eat. This feeling of being irritable, depressed, anxious, edgy and hungry sets off a second wave of eating all the wrong foods and so it continues. If you simply make a firm decision to give up refined carbohydrates for unrefined, low glycaemic-index foods, your cravings will melt away.

## Bored, frustrated, stressed

Wanting to eat when technically you're not short of fuel is purely psychological. Birds feather-pick or eat their own eggs when they are bored or stressed. Frustration and habit are other reasons for wanting to eat for the sake of it, as we simply have too little to do and too much available food. Before you say that you've got plenty to do, thank you, if you compare yourself with our primitive ancestors you're positively bone idle. Their day started with a trek for water and the hunt for food, then there was the washing, making clothes from hides, building fires and so on. When the sun went down, they slept because there was nothing else they could do. We get bored because electric light has made it possible for us to be awake when our work is done, so we fill the hours with other tasks and projects, and this thing called 'time for yourself'. For most people, time for themselves means a second half of the day to spend socializing, dancing, canoeing, visiting the sick or flying model aeroplanes, but if you're housebound because the children are in bed or you've got no money or nowhere to go, eating is often just something to do. Women feel hungrier because they think they shouldn't be eating, so they try not to, and as we all know, 'trying not to' means you usually do!

## Lack of daylight

When it was dark longer during the winter months ancient man often went for more than fourteen hours without food, so he would have tried to eat as much as he could during daylight hours. Even people who don't suffer from the 'winter blues' called Seasonal Affective Disorder (SAD) can find that they crave carbohydrates in the winter. Lack of proper daylight has an effect on the brain which is just beginning to be taken more seriously. This primitive hibernation response makes us crave carbohydrates to fill up our food stocks, and I believe it affects all people who work by artificial light which your brain knows is not proper daylight.

## Trying not to eat

Food cravings also happen when you try to avoid meals. I have noted bizarre eating patterns in women who eat more in the way of snacks and nibbles and much less at mealtimes and believe that if you can somehow avoid breakfast you won't be tempted to eat later. They'll say to me, 'I only control my weight this way, because if I have a meal it makes me want to eat for the rest of the day.' But when I look at them, they're usually overweight and I want to say, 'But haven't you noticed? It's not working!'

## The territorial response

You might also find that you have no trouble avoiding food at certain times, but other times and places trigger uncontrollable eating: the tempting sandwiches at the coffee-shop for example, the cakes at the office or the crisps and nuts at the pub. You don't really want them, but they seem to be part of the routine.

This is what I call a 'territorial' habit. Ever seen a cat bring a mouse back home? She probably puts it on the same spot on your floor or your carpet every time. Cats are hunters like us, and dogs also tend to mark out their territory in ways we're all too familiar with. Animals which bury food do it in the same spots, and this is why events, places and even people will trigger off in us a desire to eat. Have coffee at the garden centre every Tuesday? You have three custard creams as well. Lunch with parents? You always eat pudding. If you're fed up and miserable right now because you can't resist food, you need to get a grip on your territorial responses and change some old triggers.

## Water Retention

Every woman knows about water retention and feeling bloated and how it ruins entire romantic weekends. Taking your favourite trousers away with you or looking forward to slipping into that special frock and then finding that you feel like a sausage squeezed into its skin – we've all got the photos to prove it. Well, I beat it and so can you. Water retention is not an illness. There's a reason for it and if you can't stand it then you can prevent it by eating right. But why do we retain water in the first place?

After the middle of your cycle, your blood volume is increasing to enable a fertilized embryo to settle into its cosy home for nine months. Blood volume also means more water, and this makes you feel bloated and 'full' and slightly tetchy as you feel bigger and fatter. The moment your period starts it all sorts itself out, the exception to this rule being teenagers who miss the odd period and women during the change who are also skipping a month or two. In these cases the hormones can't quite decide what they want to do, so blood volume ebbs and flows and you either retain water or you don't. But the weight isn't fat! So don't keep getting on those scales until you've had your period because you'll only get depressed and panicky.

Drinking more water does NOT cause you to retain it. It flushes through what you already have and it gets rid of all kinds of nasty build-ups and constipation. If you feel big and tight you don't want to add to it by having a lot of food backed-up inside you. Sorry to be indelicate, but there's no other way of putting it. Drink extra water and you'll be flushing that system through quite happily, and I'll guarantee you'll feel much better than you do now.

Your fluid levels are carefully regulated by minerals. Sodium and potassium are essential minerals. Basically, sodium stops fluids being lost and potassium stops water being retained. Your body contains about 100g of sodium and 125g of potassium and they work in partnership, the potassium helping your kidneys to get rid of excess sodium. There is hardly ever a danger of sodium being too low except where there has been excessive sweating or water lost through crash dieting, fasting or over-use of diuretic tablets. Jockeys spring to mind as an example, because they have to weigh in at a particular weight in order to earn a living, so losing weight – any sort of weight – fast is the name of the game for them. However, the consequences of sodium depletion are not nice, as ex-jockey and racing commentator Richard Pitman explained.

I had a race that afternoon and was over four kilos over the limit. I started wasting [a racing term for losing weight] early in the day with a long sauna, but lost only about two kilos. I'd been given some diuretic tablets by a Harley Street weight-loss specialist, and he'd topped up the treatment with a massive injection. We went off to the gallops pretty early that morning prior to the journey to the race meeting, and I had to get off my horse for a pee every five minutes. I neither ate nor drank that morning for fear of pushing the weight back up, and I set off for the long journey at midday.

I stopped about a dozen times on the way, but when I arrived and was weighed I'd lost the four kilos and I went ahead. For most of the way I couldn't see, and I only hung on to the horse through sheer adrenalin – I was totally weak. I actually won the race, and as I was led into the enclosure the energy completely deserted me. I didn't dismount, I just slid off the saddle and onto the ground in front of the horse's owner. I felt so terrible I was hallucinating, and I daresay my blood sugar was rock bottom too. Needless to say I drank two cups of tea, ate normally for a day and didn't go for a pee once. When I weighed myself again I'd gained the four kilos back!

You might wonder why I've chosen this story when your water retention problem is due to hormonal activity, but only jockeys consistently go through this hell and lose so many kilos of body weight through water alone, and they do it with diuretic tablets or by sweating in a sauna. Although losing water deliberately like this is unwise it is part of the racing culture. Don't abuse your body in this way with water tablets, whether you buy them over the counter or are prescribed them by your doctor. You can easily deal with water. Restoring the balance is essential, which is why sports drinks contain salt. If you get severely dehydrated because of heat or exercise, the better and cheaper bet would be to have some plain water with a little fresh fruit juice for sweetness, and a small pinch of salt.

## Bloating

Bloating isn't an attractive word, but it's the bane of most women's lives, and the most common problem in my newspaper mailbag. It's not so much a problem of being fat as feeling fat, a monumental insult to a girl who spends her time being careful about what she eats and how much she exercises.

Strange though it might seem, it is the very acts of dieting, restricting food and being careful not to eat, which exacerbate the problems of tightness and abdominal wind. The sensation that, try as you might, you just can't hold yourself in is depressing and frustrating. I wrote a book entirely dedicated to the subject entitled *5 Days to a Flatter Stomach* and I was astounded at how many people wrote to me afterwards to thank me for the advice. It is so simple too: it's not so much what you eat but how and when you eat. You don't stop eating certain foods but you eat them at a different time of the day from when you might normally have them. You cut out certain chemicals and natural foods known to cause wind, and you get a grip on constipation. In five days a miraculous transformation takes place and your stomach is suddenly flatter and under control. The added benefit of this quick fix is a purely psychological one, but I'm all for that. Feeling slimmer makes you act slimmer, makes you stand taller and tighten your belt a notch or two. Confidence is your greatest ally in the war against body chaos, and in the second section of this book I am going to give you some simple but effective ideas for instantly banishing the bloat.

## Tired All the Time

This is not the same as 'endlessly exhausted', although there's a rather fine distinction. A new mother who is end-lessly exhausted is trying to get over the massive demands of pregnancy followed immediately by the demands of a baby: sleepless nights, repetitive routines, breastfeeding, shortage of nutrients and so on. Being 'tired all the time' rarely means needing to sleep. It can be related to these causes:

- Not drinking enough water.
- Not getting enough fresh air or exercise.
- Being bored, or not stimulated enough mentally at work or home – a job you know too well, even if it is a position of high responsibility, the same old friends, the same old neighbourhood, a stale marriage or relationship, no adult company at home, etc.

- The hormone progesterone – it is a sedative hormone, and when it is at its height, around the time of ovulation and for a few days afterwards, it can make you feel washed-out and 'woolly-headed'.

## Headaches

The causes of headache are so varied that it would be impossible and irresponsible of me to go into them all in enough detail here. If you suffer headaches on a regular basis, or if you have just started having bad headaches, you must see your doctor. The advice I am giving you is aimed at what most women would recognize instantly as hormonal headaches.

It is not completely clear why some women experience blinding headaches when they take the Pill or HRT or when going through the change, but they do, and they seem to be linked to both testosterone and oestrogen levels. It is not the level of oestrogen as such which seems to cause the headache but the fact that the level is falling. With women who take the type of contraceptive pill where you don't take a tablet during the week of your period, the few days before you start your next month of tablets and after bleeding has stopped can be pure hell, although many other women, of course, report no problems at all. Women during the menopause can experience the same effect as hormone levels fluctuate.

Women also have levels of the male hormone testosterone, and this hormone is responsible for sex drive and energy levels. There is a shift in hormones at the menopause and although your ovaries aren't making much oestrogen they continue to make testosterone in small quantities, which is why middle-aged women start to grow facial hair. As testosterone levels also decline this can result in a lack of sex drive, low energy levels and headaches.

# Chapter Three

# Allergies and Additives

I couldn't write a book about body chaos and not mention food allergies. It seems to me that it's no coincidence that reported cases of food allergy or intolerance have risen in line with our consumption of food which has already been partially prepared by manufacturers. I refer to ready meals and convenience food which need to have additives in order for them to keep longer than a day or two, even if those additives are as innocuous as soya flour, which is added to bread. On top of that, you have your disorganized eating habits. I apologize if this sounds like a mother teaching her naughty children some table manners, and I promise this is not my intention, but over the years I have advised countless people about simple table manners and habits which have totally revolutionized their digestive systems! You wouldn't believe it was so simple unless you tried it, but eating slowly, pausing between mouthfuls and making sure everything is thoroughly chewed are not just old-fashioned notions of eating; they encourage good digestion by doing most of the work before your food gets past your throat. So do give the old-fashioned methods a go!

Hormones come into it because of the effect they have on your moods, and moods affect your eating habits. Feeling low and irritable and fed up with yourself because of PMT or post-baby blues, can mean that you start gorging on food which you might not normally bother with. You won't just eat the worst foods, like ice cream, biscuits and chocolate, you eat great thumping mounds of them: family-sized tubs, entire tins. Is it any wonder that this complete overload of your internal organs lets you know it's not happy? A bowlful of dessert with artificial sweeteners and stabilizers is bad enough, but multiply that by the equivalent of twenty bowlfuls and you've got an additive overload which will take a couple of days to work through your system. So don't underestimate the damage you can do to your insides by overloading them with chemicals. You won't die, but they won't do you any good, either.

Your digestive organs exist only as a food processing plant. With many metres of working parts, it is hardly realistic to expect your digestion to carry on unnoticed by you. In fact irritable bowels are not necessarily a bad thing because some of the best food you can eat is designed to do just that – irritate the lining of your gut to provoke good expulsion of wastes. Bran does this, so do the hard lignins or pips found in strawberries and linseeds, among others. So try not to get too hung up about a bit of extra gas or wind when you have a healthy diet, and if you find it understandably aesthetically unacceptable when you are trying to look your best, leave out the culprit foods, or eat at different times of the day.

These are some causes of internal chaos.

## Too Many Additives

If our bodies aren't designed for refined food, they are even less well able to cope with chemicals. An additive is something which is added to or used in or on food which alters the taste, texture, shelf-life, colour, appearance or consistency of a food. More important – it is something in a food which you wouldn't eat on its own. You might also believe that a food label proclaiming, 'No artificial additives', 'Free from additives', or even, 'No preservatives', means what it says, but some foods don't have to be labelled this way because they are considered fresh. For example, animals or fish may have been given chemicals in their feed but the public does not have to be told.

### What Do They Do To Me?
- Cause gasiness, flatulence.
- Abdominal pain.
- Diarrhoea.
- Constipation.

### Where Do I Find Them?
- Sorbitol (E420): an artificial sweetener which is also a harmless, mild laxative used in many products.
- The artificial colour known as 'burnt sugar' or 'caramel' is added to numerous products which would otherwise be pale or grey, and is also found in: beer, colas, biscuits, crisps, bread, pickles, sauces, soups, ready meals, chocolates.
- Guar gum (E412) and xanthan gum (E415): used as thickeners in desserts and low-calorie yoghurts.
- Carageenan (E407): an emulsifier used widely in quick-set jellies, milkshakes, biscuits, pastries, sausages and meat pies. It is a laxative and causes wind.
- E431 polyoxyethylene: an emulsifier used in bread. It is also known to be slightly laxative, and the resulting 'rumbly tummy' is reported by women as a bloating effect.

There are more, but I'm sure you get my drift. Chemicals and additives shouldn't be in food and they have no place in your body. After all, bread is treated to keep it fresh for a fortnight – but why would you want that when you can freeze it or buy a fresh roll when you want one?

If you are interested in knowing more about additives, the book *Understanding Additives* published by Hodder and Stoughton for the Consumers' Association is a compulsive read! Here's an everyday example of a small pot of dessert which you wouldn't even notice eating, but which contains more additives than food:

**Sainsbury's Too Good to be True 95 per cent fat-free lemon mousse**

| Contents derived from food | Other contents |
| --- | --- |
| yoghurt | thickener |
| modified maize starch | emulsifiers |
| sugar | colour: curcumin |
| dextrose | disodium diphosphate |
| lemons | flavourings |
| vegetable fat | artificial sweetener |
| pork gelatine | stabilizer |
| lactose | lactic acid esters of mono- |
| cream | and di-glycerides of fatty acids |
| guar gum | |

So here is a product with ten sources of food and seven additives to make the whole thing work. It is a good example of something which couldn't exist without the additives.

You can avoid chemicals by buying organic products and they needn't work out expensive. If you cut out snacks you're automatically saving money, and the fact is, if you eat less it'll cost less. Spend a little of what you save on organic produce.

### 'It's So Hard When I'm Always in a Rush!'

I know it's hard, and there's no short cut to this one. If you were ill and your doctor gave you a medication which required a lot of undressing and sleeping on your side and other inconveniences, you'd still do it rather than continue feeling unwell. And is it really so hard? It is not time-consuming to eat different food. It is not time-consuming to sit down rather than stand up. I grant you, washing dishes takes longer than chucking a takeaway carton in the bin, but where has that got you so far? People always overestimate the length of time it takes to do something, and rarely think of the benefits. Being in a rush means you're doing too much and not organizing yourself properly. Get control, plan meals and put them into some kind of order. You won't be sorry.

## Allergies and Sensitivities

*'I get bloated, feel nauseous and lethargic after some meals, and I think I'm sensitive to wheat or dairy products. It's making me blow up like a balloon.'*

As the years roll by, you tend to become more sensitive to your body. It's just a fact of life. You've taken it for granted up to now, but subtle changes are beginning to show. Climbing the social or career ladder, serious relationships or break-ups all point to a time of more introspection about yourself and your looks. It goes without saying that all this time your body's been changing in ways so subtle you weren't aware of them. Shifting hormone patterns mean that by your mid to late thirties the slide towards menopause has started, but the new fad is to blame physical problems on an allergy. True allergies are rare. So what's the difference between an allergy, and an adverse reaction to food?

### Sensitivity or aversion

This tends to be a reaction or emotional response to a food rather than something caused by the food itself – such as the response to meat by a vegetarian. In blind testing when the foods are disguised, there is no response.

## Food intolerance

This describes a physiological reaction to a food which is not an immune response, such as a reaction to spices, caffeine, etc. It is usually a response to a chemical in a food.

## Food allergy

An over-reaction of your body's immune system in response to a protein in the trigger food. The common triggers are: shellfish, milk, nuts, eggs, soya bean curd. Symptoms can include a tight chest, breathing difficulties, nettle rash, runny nose, etc. and occasionally, as can be the case with a nut allergy, the outcome is fatal.

## When Is It an Allergy – and When Is It Something Else?

### Case history 1: allergy or greed?

Louise would go from breakfast until 6 p.m. without much to eat, then come home to prepare a meal. She would regularly devour half a French stick the minute she got home, and two slices of toast later. When she got wind and cramps she put it down to wheat intolerance.

### The true problem?
Fresh-baked bread devoured like a gannet is enough to cause anybody severe cramps and fatigue! You are suffering from a system overload caused by eating a lot of bread on an empty stomach. Eating too much, too quickly and after a long gap is bound to cause cramps and nausea.

## Case history 2: allergy or too much dieting?

Davina complained of breathlessness after eating dairy products. She claimed to feel better if she drank water and ate fruits and vegetables.

### The true problem?
Davina got checked out by a doctor who found low iron levels which cause breathlessness. She was also looking for an excuse to avoid what she thought were fatty foods.

## Case history 3: allergy or stress?

Sheila found her heart would often race after meals, causing panic attacks. She blamed meat, as it only happened on a Friday when she had a regular steak lunch with her husband.

### The true problem?
Friday was also accounts day, and Sheila worked a full, stomach-churning morning without a break. Meat is hard to digest unless chewed properly, but a change to shepherd's pie which, being made from minced meat requires less chewing, and a mid-morning milky coffee did the trick.

## Case history 4: allergy or too many chemicals?

Theresa grew up in the country, and boasted of having the constitution of an ox. A few months after moving to London, she had bouts of bloatedness, indigestion, intestinal wind and loose bowels. Theresa blamed an allergy to certain types of fruit and bread, as it only seemed to happen when she ate her lunchtime sandwiches and fruit salad.

### The true problem?
At home, Theresa had eaten a cooked lunch and only ever ate her mother's home-made bread. Shop-bought sandwiches made with commercial bread contain soya flour and

flour improvers, both of which cause intestinal gas, and her fruit salad was sweetened with sorbitol, a safe sweetener which nonetheless can cause wind. By 5 p.m. her stomach felt tight and uncomfortable, but a return to meat and vegetables for lunch and bread made without additives soon resolved her problem.

## Your Plan of Action

- Eat slowly.
- Don't leave longer than three hours between meals.
- Eat fresh food.
- Follow the Beat Your Body Chaos Diet on page 187 or the wheat-free diet on page 210 for a fortnight, then gradually introduce your old favourites one by one.
- Stop smoking. If you have to smoke, have your last cigarette an hour before a meal and don't have another one until an hour afterwards. This helps to slow gut transit time.

# Keeping a Food Diary

Recording what, where and when you eat and drink might seem to be self-obsessed, cumbersome and a nuisance to begin with, but it has been shown that people who keep tabs on intake usually succeed in conquering their weight. When I take on a new client, he or she has to keep a food diary for a whole two weeks before we can even get started. This covers a couple of weekends and should include any special difficulties like birthdays or a day out. Invariably when they hand it in to me they remark that they never realized either how much they ate or how bad their diet was.

You simply write down everything that passes your lips for two weeks. When I ask clients to do this for me they often try to impress me by not writing down exact quantities or by hiding really bad habits, but I'm not interested in just their food intake but the pattern of their eating. Many people eat very little all day, for example, then graze all evening. Others eat on the dot of certain times and never in between (though this is rare), or they might only ever eat three or four different meals. I look at the frequency of fruit servings, or vegetables, or diet drinks, and it's common to find very little fruit and vegetables but many diet drinks taken in the daytime to stave off hunger pangs. I need to see the pattern and discuss it with the client, because it is only by identifying why and where you ate something that you can begin to understand why you might be having problems with weight, energy levels and even headaches or eczema.

This is what a food diary might look like:

**Date:**

| Time | What Eaten | What Doing |
|---|---|---|
| 7.45 a.m. | 1 slice toast, no butter, 1 tsp marmalade. Cup of tea. | Standing in kitchen. |
| 10.15 a.m. | 2 custard creams, diet Coke. | Sitting at desk. |
| 10.25 a.m. | 1 fruit pastille. | Friend offered. |
| 1.20 p.m. | Tuna baguette, Müllerice, 1 apple, 2 cups machine coffee. | Sitting at desk. |
| 4.05 p.m. | Diet Coke, 1 custard cream. | Sitting at desk. |
| 6.00 p.m. | 2 carrot sticks, 2 pretzels, 1 glass wine, 1 diet Coke. Half slice white bread with pate from making children's sandwiches. | Preparing dinner. |

| | | |
|---|---|---|
| 7.10 p.m. | Breaded chicken portion, carrots, peas, few chips, second helping of 2 spoons peas, portion chips, scoop ice cream. Finished off son's ice cream. Glass water, glass wine. Small portion tinned rice pudding with jam. Half Twix bar. Coffee. | With family at table. |
| 9.35 p.m. | Glass wine, few Pretzels, apple. | Watching TV. |
| 10.45 p.m. | 2 spoons leftover rice pudding. | In kitchen waiting for kettle. |

## What You Do Next

- Identify 'thoughtless' food like the odd polo mint, swig of wine or whatever. Write them down.
- Identify the number of meals which seem to be repeated, such as Weetabix every day for breakfast, a cheese sandwich every day for lunch, etc.
- Count the pieces of fruit you consume over seven days. It should be no fewer than twenty-one.
- Count the number of vegetable or salad portions. It should be no fewer than twenty-one. A 'portion' counts as each spoonful of vegetables, including frozen vegetables. A mixed salad would count as two portions.
- Count the number of drinks (non-alcoholic) you have. It should add up to 2.25 litres a day.
- Count the alcohol units. You should have no more than fourteen if you are a woman, twenty-one if a man.
- Add up your milk consumption. It should be a 500 ml of skimmed milk a day. Count a portion of cereal as 125 ml.
- Try to even out the amounts of food you have at each meal. Many people say that if they start the day eating, they will continue to overeat all day. This will happen at first, but it rarely continues. As soon as you know you have another meal coming up in a few hours' time, the temptation to eat too much vanishes. You should be eating much less in the evening, and a little more for breakfast and lunch.

This is the basis of a better diet. See the Beat Your Body Chaos Diet page 187 or write your own – and stick to it!

## Your Polluted Body!

Body chaos can also be caused by pollution. Your hormones have a job to do and sometimes they do it when all the odds are stacked up against them. Take melatonin for example. You'll remember that this is the hormone which switches on at night to tell you to go to sleep, but what do we do when it signals its arrival? Have another cup of coffee, light a cigarette, or go out to a noisy club where we intend staying awake for another four or five hours! Our insulin levels are strained to the limit with high-carbohydrate takeaways and chocolate, and adrenalin pours out at inappropriate hours of the day and night as we queue up for taxis, have arguments or get wheel-clamped. But by far the worst strain for us are oxidants.

Oxidants come in various forms, but the ones you need to be concerned about are free radicals, and the older you get the more likely you are to be attacked by these trouble-making, roaming oxygen reactions. Yes, the very stuff which gives us life can also help to take it away. Becoming oxidized is rather like going rancid – like a steak that has been around too long – because free radicals attack the fatty parts of cell membranes. So what are free radicals and can you stop them attacking you?

We are all made up of billions of cells. Inside those cells are molecules and inside the molecules are electrons. The important feature of electrons is that they like to go around in pairs. When your body is being attacked by poisons, the electrons get separated from their twin so they go around desperately trying to find another electron to pair with, so they take somebody else's twin and that leaves him without, and so on and so on. This continual search leads to a cascade of reactions, so like anything on the rampage you have these destructive electrons causing cell death. On an everyday level this causes skin ageing: the worst scenario is cancer.

## What Causes This Separation?

Your body is being attacked by poisons – from food and from the atmosphere. Here are some of the danger signs:

- Living in a city.
- Sunbathing or not protecting your body from ultra-violet rays.
- Smoking – or breathing somebody else's smoke.
- A lot of barbecued food.
- Processed food.
- Too much alcohol.
- Stress – cortisol can make your immune system weak.

## Can I Do Anything About It?

Yes. Your body can mount a brilliant defence against free-radical attack in the same way that you can be immunized against a virus. These are called anti-oxidant defences, and they come from vitamins A, C, E and the mineral selenium. If you are at greater risk because you live near a motorway, smoke or work outdoors, you might need more of these vitamins.

On page 179 I outline a good plan of action to help you

harness your defences against attack. After all, it would be a shame if all your hard work in beating mood swings, PMS, water retention and weight gain was rendered useless because you get ill from too much sunbathing!

# Chapter Four

# What Is Your Body Made Of?

How would you describe your body? Is it hard, flabby, saggy, lean or lumpy? Most women want a body which is toned and taut, but muscle is soft tissue which means that if it is not contracted in a movement, it is soft and easily mistaken for fat. For example, your latissimus dorsi muscles which move your arm out to the side can look like fat if they are well-developed. You can go down a dress size and be euphoric about inch loss around your stomach area when in fact it's your buttock muscles which have dropped, making your overall inch measurement on your hips much smaller. A bout of healthy cycling can mean your jeans are suddenly tighter as your muscle fibres increase in number and again, I'll get frantic letters from readers asking why they've suddenly got so fat. They haven't.

Your body doesn't come with an instruction manual, and while it's probably wise to understand what it's made of and how to look after it you might feel that it's like your car and you'd rather pay someone to look under the bonnet for you than actually have to go to the trouble of going to engine maintenance classes. That's fair enough, but whereas you can trade in an old car, washing machine or lawnmower and never set eyes on them again, if your body goes wrong you're stuck with the consequences. I'm constantly amazed that most people simply haven't a clue about the way they are constructed. So your first priority is to learn what you're made of, and why this can make such a difference to your hormones, weight and looks.

## Fat

We think of all fat as being the same but in a slim woman, about 10 per cent of her total body weight is what is called 'essential fat'. A man has just 3 per cent. In women fat is located in:

- The breasts
- Around the ovaries
- As 'packing' for vital organs
- Insulation for nerves
- A fat 'pad' which seats the eye in its socket

Storage fat or 'adipose tissue' as it is more properly termed, consists almost entirely of fat-filled cells held in a loose mesh of fibrous tissue which is supplied by blood vessels and nerves. It is found packed around your abdominal organs, between bundles of muscles and layered under your skin. The difference between men and women in fat storage is that women keep more under their skin and men carry it in a 'paunch'.

Storage fat is what happens to calories when you don't need them. You are either eating too much or exercising too little but whichever it is, the excess energy gets laid down as emergency fuel stores. Your body has enough storage fat to enable you to stay alive for many weeks without food, or to exercise for 5–10 days, depending on what sort of exercise you are doing. You have approximately 35,000,000,000 fat cells, each containing 45mcg of fat. As people become obese these cells can store double this amount of fat, giving rise to the as yet unproven theory that people who have lost huge amounts of weight – say more than half their body weight – have fat cells which crave refuelling because they are bigger. I'll talk about this again in the section on 'Leptin', but it would certainly seem to answer the question about why some people simply cannot control their appetites for long, especially in the case of so-called 'yo-yo' dieters. However, it is not enough to blame fat cells for your weight gain when your eating habits might need to be reassessed.

Brown fat is tissue which is present in babies, young children and hibernating animals, and it prevents you from freezing to death. It metabolizes fats at a high rate by generating heat, and is sometimes known as a 'weight thermostat'.

## Android or Gynoid?

Most of us are either android or gynoid body types. An android type has slender legs and tends not to gain weight on her thighs or buttocks but she might have a thick waist. Being an android shape is fine if you want to make the most of a slim lower half but it can have quite a high health risk. It is known that android fat distribution increases the risk of coronary heart disease, and some of this is explained in the section 'stress and weight gain' (page 32). As this fat is broken down for emergency fuel, the fatty acids in the blood rise, and there is a risk of clogged arteries leading to high blood pressure.

Gynoid fat distribution on the other hand, leads to the classic 'pear shape', with fat deposits on thighs, hips and buttocks. This type of fat responds to the female hormones which make it easier to be broken down for general fuel and for pregnancy rather than for stress, and this is why it tends to stay on the lower body rather than entering the bloodstream. Good news for your health maybe, but not so brilliant for those slimline thighs!

At the age of eight, boys and girls have something like 16–18 per cent body fat. By the age of seventeen during the adolescent growth spurt, girls increase body-fat percentage to about 25 per cent, while boys decrease to around 12–15 per cent. By their early twenties, girls have usually increased body-fat percentage to 26–29 per cent, and between the ages of thirty to sixty, body-fat percentage increases steadily, at a rate of 1.5–2 per cent a decade.

## Is There Anything Good About Being a Little Overweight?

Yes and no. In your fat you have an enzyme called aromatase which converts androgens (male hormones) to oestrogen, so if you have extra fat you have higher levels of oestrogen. Now these higher levels can actually do some good. They can, for example, protect you against osteoporosis, because it is known that for all women, and particularly at the meno-pause when oestrogen begins to dwindle, low oestrogen levels can mean a risk of brittle bones. On the other hand, being fat and having higher oestrogen can be a negative factor because of the risk of breast cancer. On the whole though, the negative side of being fat outweighs the positive because you can have other problems like painful joints, and the psychological difficulties of not being able to fit into your clothes or wear the things you really want to wear. So it's always better to keep excess fat in check, in the same way that it's better not to be too thin.

## Could My Fat Stores Run Out?

In theory, yes, but it's not the fat loss which causes death but the breakdown of protein, which is the next stage. This is very damaging as your body literally starts to eat its own tissues. This happens to anybody in an extreme state of starvation and it doesn't need too vivid an imagination to work out that this is a very nasty end indeed.

The other circumstance where fat stores could run out is in fact not an accurate way of putting it. The fat remains but your body cannot get at it. This happens during long-distance runs and similar feats of endurance where the glucose in the muscles has run out. Fitness classes refer rather glibly to 'fat-burning exercise', but fat is not suddenly brought out as fuel the minute your heart rate increases. It is the great length of the period of exercise which results in fat being brought into play, which is why a long day's general activity is worth more for your weight and figure than a fast, hard game of squash.

## Muscle

Apart from cardiac muscle and the smooth muscles which contract of their own accord such as in the gut and in the lining of the womb, the muscles you will be concerned with are the skeletal muscles.

These muscles are attached to bones, and you could not move without them. In my *Monica's Fabulous Body Plan* mini-books, I describe the muscles and the movements which produce a particular effect on your figure: for example, running is a good exercise, but it won't improve your arms or chest; swimming won't help your calves, and so on. It is vital that every woman learns about her muscle structure and how to exercise each part of her body to maintain a balance.

There are tens of thousands of fibres in each muscle and weight gain should always be achieved by increasing muscle size not gaining fat. Muscles grow in size when they are asked to work harder by lifting heavier weights, which is why weight training can produce some dramatic effects.

## Bones

Your skeleton is a finely-engineered structure with the strength of steel. It is a tough foundation on to which everything else in your body is attached or fixed, but unlike steel it is light enough for you to be able to carry it around. It is true that some people have such exceptionally heavy bones that they can use them as an excuse for being several kilos overweight, and there are some pretty large-framed people about, just as there are some very petite ones. Bones are more important than we realize, and it's only when a woman has lost her strength to brittle-bone disease that she discovers just how valuable they were. Bones cannot be repaired once they have become brittle. It is up to us to look after them, and up to parents to see to it that their children are encouraged to walk, to eat and drink calcium-rich foods, and to see their skeleton as the most important foundation they have. It never ceases to amaze me that we have our children inoculated against diseases they probably wouldn't get anyway, shield them from dangers that are equally as unlikely, yet drive them to school and let them eat junk food because it's giving them what they are asking for. It is tantamount to neglect.

Here are a few bone facts which all of us should take seriously:

- Peak bone strength is around twenty to thirty years of age. After this there is nothing you can do to strengthen your bones any further.
- Bones need 'loading' – or put under stress through weight-bearing exercise like walking and running, and this increases their density to make them incredibly hard, strong and thick. Exercise which bears your weight, like swimming, is not so good for bones.
- Very intensive exercise is damaging to bones, especially if you have a very low body weight. Put simply, if you are training every day using 2,500

calories of energy and only eating 1,000 calories, your bones will not have the calories they need for repair.

- If you go under 50 kilos in weight, your hormones won't function properly. This might mean missed periods because your body won't make oestrogen. Without oestrogen your bones might suffer the same effects of ageing as you would see in someone of fifty or sixty, who had gone through the menopause.

- The hormone oestrogen keeps bones strong and healthy. If you are going through the menopause, don't take HRT willy-nilly just because your GP says it will protect you against osteoporosis, because you might not be in any danger – so ask for a bone scan. I did, and my bones proved to be 14 per cent above normal – which is just about the most cheering thing I'd heard all year.

# Chapter Five

# It Must Be In My Genes!

One thing none of us can do anything about is change our parents. We can inherit some pretty good characteristics from them, endless legs and fabulously lustrous hair, but also some quite depressing ones, a long chin, hooked nose, big ears. Hormonal tendencies can also be inherited, so if you want to know if your menopause will start early, ask your mother about hers.

Mind you, I have always thought that some period problems are learned behaviour. Observe your mother or sister writhing in agony every twenty-eight days and you might just think it's normal; my casual research has told me that in homes where bodily functions are taboo subjects, girls report little trouble with pain. It's not that they don't experience it, it's just that they might not think it worth mentioning.

So big busts run in families, so do thick legs, fat backs and double chins. But does fat run in families, or is it something far deeper than that? Family tendencies also demonstrate themselves in eating and exercise habits, and the type of company you keep, and Nikki is an example.

When Nikki was seventeen she weighed 76 kilos (12 stone). Her mother and father are also overweight, as are her sister and aunt. Nikki assumed that her size was a family tendency, and she felt depressed and powerless. This led her to lose pride in herself because she felt there was no remedy. She was facing a downward spiral of despair and neglect of herself. She said that there was no point in trying to diet because her fatness was in her genes.

When babies are born, they look to their mothers for everything. They copy what she does, and if their early months are spent in the arms of a mother who never goes anywhere, this is all they know. Fat parents tend to avoid brisk walks, might drive their children to school and base enjoyable activities around meals, snacks and drinks. Nikki had been brought up in this atmosphere and was simply copying her parents' behaviour, resulting in a body type like theirs. All she had to do to change her appearance was adopt a more active lifestyle and take charge of her eating.

Now nineteen, Nikki has taken control of her eating and her weight has fallen from 101 kilos (16 stone) at the age of fifteen to her current weight of 57 kilos (9 stone). Her problem was a large extended family, with most meals lovingly prepared by her grandmother. So how did she go about it? Here's her story:

I used to spend a lot of time round my nan's because my mum was out at work. She always had a chocolate treat for me, and being a child I obviously loved having as many sweets as I could. I gained a lot of weight which I suppose bothered me, but I thought it would sort itself out.

As time went on and I got into my teens, I noticed that everyone at school was talking about weight, and I realized how fat I was. I knew that I was stressed a lot of the time, and I think most of it was because of the home situation. Mum felt guilty about working, I felt I always had to please my nan by eating whatever she'd cooked for me, and in a way I was always ravenously hungry, as if food was making up for something. At home my mum and I talked about nothing else but weight! I'd cut back for a few days, then my mum would worry that she was pressuring me, so she gave me a cream cake to calm the atmosphere. It was comfort food that worked in reverse! At the time it would take away the tension and I'd think, 'Well, this is just how I am.' But deep inside I'd be miserable. I was picked on all the time at school so I'd go home and eat even more. I got so stressed I ended up in hospital, then I went to a special school for a while.

Then my nan died. I was upset of course, but it was a sort of liberation from having to please her all the time. I couldn't afford slimming clubs so I started by not having as many chips, then one cake instead of two. I also started an evening snack, because up until then whenever I tried to lose weight I ate as little as I could and tried not to eat after 6 p.m. I just got ravenous. Eating a small snack about 9 o'clock made me feel a lot better.

I know that a lot of people say that encouraging teenagers to diet will spark off an eating disorder, but they just don't understand the mental torture of hating every bit of your body, and feeling trapped by it. I lost a lot of weight, but it certainly wasn't all plain sailing, and I still have lapses.

One of the biggest challenges was managing my family, and I think this comes back to whether fatness is in your genes. My mum and my nan always gave us money for chips and that's just the way our family was. I can't ever remember seeing fruit or salad in our kitchen – the chip pan is more or less permanently on the go. I feel as if I need to go to a school that'll teach me to plan meals and shop and cook in a healthy way, because I haven't a clue. I'm not blaming my mum or nan, but I see now how I got this weight problem. Part of it was the general way we did things in our house, and then someone told me that stress can make you fat because of all the adrenalin which makes you want to eat. I can certainly identify with that! It's been hard, but I think you just have to be aware of the moments when you'd have rushed to the biscuit tin and just say, 'Stop!' Now I do something else instead.

You have to sit down with your mum and tell her how unhappy you are, but don't make it a whinge or a complaint otherwise she'll get hurt about the way she's been bringing you up. What I've learned though, is that my size had nothing to do with my parents and everything to do with the habits in our house. Now I'm slim I've got a really normal figure like anyone else, not the spare tyre or 'family' double chin I was told I'd have for the rest of my life. I know I'm young, but I wish I'd eaten more healthily and sensibly sooner, or that someone had taken better trouble to see I didn't get so fat.

**Make no mistake about it – giving your children fried foods and cakes is not a sign of neglect. Many loving, caring**

parents feed their children the best way they can, and families are no more caring just because there's a healthy salad on the table. Neglect happens when a parent knowingly feeds the children a second-rate poor diet out of idleness or thrift, but the child must take charge of herself when she's old enough and learn how to adapt what she's learned at home for the future.

## Is It Wrong to Encourage Dieting?

There's nothing wrong with wanting to be slim. I want to be slim. It's no worse than wanting to keep your hair a certain style or preferring jeans to skirts. If you can see your shape as simply another element of the style you've chosen for yourself, you are keeping a sense of proportion. But weight and size are two different things and, in my view, the attractiveness of a girl lies in how she is put together. A tiny figure with a slim pair of legs and boyish hips – the sort we all secretly wish we had – can look unattractive if they are topped by a hard face. A beautiful face with a laughing smile is spoilt if you can hardly drag your hips out of the chair. Looking as if you care about your body is about more than where the needle stops on the scales. You must start caring about the impression you make, and if you look as if your spare time is spent watching TV with a takeaway and chips, you can't be surprised if prospective employers think twice about you. Yes, it's the person inside who really counts, but if your external appearance suggests inactivity and gluttony or secret bingeing and vomiting you can hardly blame people for not wanting to hang around to discover your inner depths!

Looking healthy is a prerequisite of attracting good responses from people, so don't be railroaded into staying on an unhealthy, childish diet. Sweets might taste nice, but they aren't grown-up food and they contain little in the way of good nutrients.

## Stop Weighing Yourself All the Time!

Does weight matter?

Yes, weight matters when it's the difference between being too fat or too thin. Weight matters if you've suddenly lost it for no good reason – a good reason being that you've suffered a tragedy or are stressed or have had a sickness bug. But other, sudden losses in weight which you cannot put down to a known cause can include early signs of diabetes. This could happen because your sugar levels are out of control and your body is desperately trying to flush out the excess. You would not be long in reaching a diagnosis however, because you would have a raging thirst, weight loss as I said, and you would be running to the loo incessantly. So if you have lost weight without these symptoms, don't worry, but do go and get a check up.

The more common blight on most people's lives is getting fat. It is one thing to go on holiday, over-indulge for a fortnight and come back half a stone heavier, and quite another matter to live as you have always lived and suddenly find you are two sizes larger. This is the thrust of my bulging mailbag each week from readers of my magazine column. 'What have I done wrong?' people cry, or, 'Please help! I've had a trim figure all my life and suddenly it's all gone to pot!' Of course people don't suddenly gain a stone. What they mean is that they've just noticed it and they're understandably shocked and distressed. It's like suddenly noticing how wrinkled you've become round the eyes, or how you've got jowls. It can't have happened overnight, it's just that you weren't used to studying your jawline. Monitoring your weight without becoming obsessed is plain common sense if you want to avoid these shocks, but how fat is fat – and how thin is thin?

Man wasn't designed to carry huge amounts of fat to slow him down, and being overweight makes you breathless, puts a strain on your knees, hips and back and robs you of a good figure. The old 'big-boned' theory is correct in that you can have a bigger and wider frame than somebody else, but bones don't weigh a lot. In fact a heavy skeleton would be a significant design fault, so bones tend to be strong but very light. Strong and dense bones add somewhat to your weight compared with fragile, porous or brittle bones, but this is only to the good and it doesn't account for massive fluctuations in weight, nor account for a weight gain or loss of several kilos, much as it might suit you to imagine so! So what about being too thin? How would you know if you were underweight?

It is actually quite easy to know, because your periods will stop. They stop, because, as you remember from the earlier section about adolescence, although Mother Nature wants us to have babies she doesn't want you to get pregnant at the expense of your own life. So you are prevented from getting pregnant by not ovulating, ovulation being stimulated by oestrogen levels which are in turn stimulated by your levels of fat. Generally speaking, once an adult woman's weight falls below about 50 kilos her periods will stop, and you can be sure that you are then classed as underweight.

Don't judge your appearance by your weight. Don't regard weight gain as failure and loss as success. If you lost weight through dehydration or illness, you'd hardly have been successful at anything. Your body weight is the result of a mixture of many components, not the least of which is the weight of the food you have just eaten. Anyway, gaining weight can be the making of some people. Body changes happen for all sorts of reasons, and sometimes you scratch your head in wonder at why your weight's changed. So I'd prefer to talk about gaining or losing fat, not weight, because it's the fat in your body which indicates your state of health and fitness. Here are examples of weight changes which are not related to fat:

- Getting a new hobby which requires physical effort, buying a dog which needs walking, learning to ride a horse, etc. All these activities increase muscle fibres which weigh a fifth more again than fat.

- Changing to a job where you might be lifting, pushing, reaching. This can increase muscle size and mean slight weight gain, although this might also be cancelled out by using up extra calories!

- Worry and stress – you might not be aware of it, but you will be sweating a little bit more and can lose as much as an extra 2.25kg a day through fluid loss.

- Illness with diarrhoea or sickness. Obviously as food and fluid leave your body at a faster rate than normal this means you weigh less. Sorry to be indelicate, but if you vomit an entire meal, you've just lost 1kg of body weight – but your body will look exactly the same!

- Giving blood – a 560ml of blood weighs about 750g – quick weight loss but not of fat!

- And finally, weight gain through directly eating food which is not the same as fat loss through excess calories. If you're the person who always claims she only has to look at a slice of chocolate cake to gain 2kg you might not be far out. As an example, you're going out for a meal, and you weigh yourself just before setting off – a comforting 60.3 kilos exactly. In the next two hours you eat:

- rump steak – 226g
- jacket potato – 170g
- plate of vegetables – 113g
- glass of red wine – 141g
- two glasses of water – 340g
- fruit salad – 226g
- small portion cheese – 56g
- crackers – 56g
- three cups of coffee – 255g

Total weight of food and drink =1.583kg

Assuming that you haven't needed to go to the loo, if you step straight back on the scales you'll now weigh 62 kilos, but is this true weight gain? Of course not. 568ml of liquid such as water or beer weighs 510g, so drinking several litres results in the appropriate weight gain, cancelled out of course by trips to the loo. Alcohol is a diuretic, so you are in fact losing through excretion slightly more fluids than you are taking in, which can mean dehydration. This throughput is considerably slowed down if you are also eating, and as food carries a lot of water you are also adding valuable fluids to your body when you eat as well as drink.

So when should you weigh yourself? No more than once a month if your weight is usually quite steady, and never in the week before your period. You need to get an idea of general trends rather than getting hung up on one reading, so weigh yourself at the same time of day, without clothes. If you notice that your weight is always slightly higher, this is a trend. If you are starting a weight-loss diet, weigh yourself every week.

## What Am I Doing Wrong?

Sometimes despite your best efforts, you just don't understand why your regime isn't working. Here are some of the common problems.

### Weight Gain and Anti-depressants

Anti-depressants are not fattening in themselves, but by calming your levels of anxiety they will affect your calorie-burning rates. There is something called 'Non Exercise Activity Thermogenesis' which refers to calorie-burning which is not generated by physical activity. Fidgeting, shivering, getting up and down, fussing about and so on, can burn anything from an extra 100 to 500 calories a day. In fact, we often associate 'nervy' people with being very thin. If part of your problem has been anxiety, this could have affected your appetite – you've eaten less and worried more – and it is these few hundred calories here and there which can make a depressed or anxious person lose weight while they are ill. Because anti-depressants calm you, they affect your metabolic rate. Instead of losing, you are keeping these few hundred calories which can quickly become several thousand, and it only takes a month for a few grams (a kilo) to be gained. Not a lot, but this soon becomes a few kilos – and you then blame the pills.

If you go on to anti-depressants, be aware of this effect and make sure you are a bit more active and eat 150 calories a day less.

### Weight Gain and the Pill or HRT

Hundreds of thousands of women blame the Pill or HRT for their weight gain. They are convinced that the hormones are the cause because if they stop taking them, they lose weight. But it cannot be caused by the hormones themselves because the only way fat is stored is if you go into negative energy balance, in other words if you eat more calories than you expend in activity. Hormones themselves are not fattening; neither are vitamins. You should remember that plenty of women take HRT or the Pill and don't gain weight. You must look at all the areas of your life and see where your energy expenditure has become less, and remember that even a slight change in routine amounting to 100 calories a day – such as having a short lift in someone's car when once you walked – soon mounts up to 36,500 in a year. That's 5 kilos of excess weight! So no, you're not doing anything wrong, but you've simply not kept rigid tabs on your energy levels and food intake.

## Can't be Bothered?

We've all seen the endless magazine features on being 'forever young' or 'holding back the years'. Well, you can hold back the years and stop the clock and all the other easy phrases which are tossed out to give us hope, but you can't undo the damage once it's done unless you write an enormous cheque to a willing cosmetic surgeon. But why paper over the cracks if you don't have to? People who look good when they are older tended to start young. If you can't be bothered with your looks now, you'll wish you had later. It's not just about looking 'young' or having nice skin or a slim figure, it's about people being amazed at how good you look. It's about endless compliments and an incredibly happy outlook for the whole of your life – not just the first few years.

## But I'm Having a Good Time – I'll Worry About All That When the Time Comes!

That's like saying, 'I'm having a good time so I can't be bothered cleaning my teeth' or, 'I'm having a good time so I can't waste time washing my hair or ironing my clothes'. The two things are actually dependent on each other. You won't have a good time if you have to face your friends in dirty creased clothes or with greasy hair so you get the job done. You can't have a good time if your face is so spotty and your teeth so brown everyone laughs at you behind your back. You can't enjoy yourself if you're so shattered you have to make your excuses and go home before everyone else.

Anyway, looking after yourself is hardly laser surgery. You have to eat, so rather than a burger and chips, have a salad which you don't even have to go out for. You don't think salad's as tasty as a burger? Neither do I, but who cares if every girl in the room envies you? You can get a tan from a bottle and if you stop smoking you'll have enough money for a dozen outfits.

There is a lot of emphasis these days on having everything you want in life and enjoying every moment, but sacrifices have to be made. Nobody ever became an Olympic athlete without hours of training, nobody ever qualified as a doctor without spending seven years at university. You can't get to be a world-famous singer unless you practise and practise – but there has to be a trade-off. Feeling healthy and looking good require some small sacrifices and a bit of effort, but time spent on yourself comes for free. So why not be bothered? You've nothing to lose but your looks.

# Chapter Six

# Eating Your Way Out of Chaos

## Getting Started With the Right Diet

Good nutrition is the cornerstone of a happy life. Good nutrition is the key to mastering those hormones. You might think that you already eat well, but eating is so common-place that a lot of food can pass your lips unnoticed. A meal can be a ritual, a pleasure or simply a routine, but to your body it is a lot more than that. It is an important, momentous event which promotes life or death. Like a baby who cries out to be fed, your billions of cells rely on you totally for their nourishment. Food can prevent disease, alter your moods and influence your memory. It can make you grow and bounce back after injury. Without food, these things are not possible. So how can it make any sense to deprive your body of what it needs?

## What Is a Meal?

A meal is defined as an amount of food eaten at one period of time which provides 200 calories or more. You should sit down to eat a meal and use a knife and fork, so train your-self to reject all one-food snacks which use fingers. Rejecting snacks is the best way to start a healthy diet because it doesn't deprive you of nice food at meal times. Eating proper meals is the best way to keep your weight steady because there is good evidence that the number of meals taken in a day and the amount of food eaten at one time, influences how your body uses the nutrients from those meals.

You rarely find that an entire meal passes your lips without you being able to remember it. It's the snacks and nibbles and their random nature which cause the problem, simply because their calories aren't counted. You have a bite from someone's cake, a sip of wine, a crisp from an open packet or a lick of the spoon and these are seen as free foods. In fact the calories from this sort of eating can quickly tot up to 100, which is fine as a one-off – but are they ever one-offs? In a month those calories could rise to 2,700 and the point is – were they even worth it? Did you have a fantastic, memorable time eating them?

## Starting a Very Nutritious Eating Plan

There is no such thing as a healthy food. On the face of it an apple is healthy, but if you ate nothing but apples you would get sick. A packet of crisps is not thought of as a healthy food, but if you had been living on nothing but fruit, crisps would be exactly what your body would be crying out for! So anybody considering a change of lifestyle and diet should be looking at the complete picture. A varied diet actually short-circuits the nutrition problem because it is the best way of making sure you are getting your full complement of nutrients. In many countries people eat diets which are totally different to our own, yet they manage to stay healthy and grow, so we can only assume that it is not the particular foods we eat that matters so much as the materials in those foods, which make for a balanced regime.

Most people know well enough what they should be

eating but are somehow reluctant to take the advice on board. Usually they see no reason, just as the cigarette smoker will justify her habit on the basis of the possibility that she will be one of those ninety-year-olds who have smoked for seventy years and are still going strong, or the sweet eater who sees that her teeth don't decay the minute she pops a fruit pastille into her mouth. It's hard to take advice when there seems to be no pressing reason to change, so a measure of intelligent foresight is required. Eating well isn't just about the difference between living or dying, having a disease or being in peak health. It's about the difference between feeling lousy when you wake in the morning, having a nasty scaly skin or a scalp which itches constantly, having hot, burning feet which drive you mad or endless cold bugs, and feeling so good that you embrace each day with no thoughts about your body or reminders of your health. I actually spoke to someone recently who ate a truly appalling diet of chocolate, cake, fizzy drinks and more chocolate, yet she genuinely had not suspected the link between this regime and her chronic fatigue. Did she know that five portions of fruit and vegetables a day were recommended in a healthy diet? Was she aware that she had not had a single item of fruit in a month? The answer to both these questions was 'yes', but she was young, slim and had a demanding job and a hectic social life which she assumed were responsible for her general malaise. Needless to say, a new diet transformed her life, especially leaving out all the sugar, but even so I remained shaken by her total disregard for the needs of her body.

You have to eat, so it's as easy to eat well as badly. A boiled egg, a jacket potato, a grilled steak or a roast chicken can all be cooked quickly with no preparation at all. If nobody teaches you to prepare food properly you can't be blamed, but do bone up on basic cooking skills like poaching, grilling and pan-frying, for simplicity.

# What You Need In a Good Diet

## Water: Does it Matter?

A lot of weight problems, physical problems, tiredness, depression, bloatedness, irritability and breathlessness – I could go on – are down to simply not drinking enough plain water! It is not that water affects your hormone status directly, but rather that dehydration affects your mental state, making you less inclined to activity. You can actually feel very unwell without enough fluids: light-headed, 'muzzy' and hungry, and the knock-on effects can result in worse period pains, eating problems and irritable bowels. And in case you feel that this doesn't apply to you because you never feel thirsty, you don't have to. Being short of water is not such a physical emergency that your body needs to signal its distress with a raging thirst. If you have a raging thirst however, it is serious news that your body is on its last legs.

Lack of water causes:

- constipation
- headaches
- bloated, tight stomach
- tiredness and lethargy
- dry hair
- bad breath

Aesthetically, the difference between a well-hydrated person and a dehydrated person is like the difference between a grape and a raisin, a plum and a prune, a fresh tomato and the sundried version. The dried ones are wrinkled, the fresh ones are full of water, plumped out and tempting.

- How much of me is water? About thirty-two kilos (five stone).
- How do I get more, apart from drinking? From your diet, especially from:

  fruit and vegetables which contain 18 per cent water

  milk and yoghurt which contain10 per cent water

  bread and cereals which contain 8 per cent water

  eggs, fish, meat and pulses which contain 2 per cent water
- How you lose water every day:

  | | |
  |---|---|
  | From breathing | 0.5 litres |
  | Through your skin | 0.5 litres |
  | From urine | 1.4 litres |
  | In faeces | 0.1 litres |
  | Total | 2.5 litres lost each day, which weighs 3 kilos |
- So it is incredibly important to eat regularly, not just for the food but for its water content too. A simple chicken sandwich with tomato adds an extra 17g water to your body!
- Water after exercise. There is a simple rule of thumb for rehydrating your body after exercise. You need to take in 150 per cent of what you have lost, so if you have lost a litre you must drink 1.5 litres. How do you know how much you have lost? Assume 1 litre for every hour you are exercising.

## Unrefined Carbohydrates

We are all primitive, with a primitive physiology. I find it amazing that after all these millions of years, we have hardly changed in the way we move and perform our bodily functions. Yet thousands of years ago all man had to eat was meat, berries, seeds and nuts, with the latter three only available at certain times of the year. It hardly bears thinking about that we existed on meat alone, yet this is what we were designed for. Some starches in the form of roots and tubers were presumably eaten after being cooked (starch cannot be digested if it is not cooked), but vegetables and grains as we know them were not around.

Move forward to just 150 years ago, and you get a more

sophisticated, varied diet, but still a largely unrefined one. By this time, the only refined foods were fermented alcohol and honey, and other foods were either meat, fish, vegetables and fruit or bread made with coarse wheat grains, coarse rice and so on. The only reason flour became refined was to keep the weevils out during storage, but the main point about refining is that it is relatively new to the human body, and not something it is used to coping with. Refining also takes out about 80 per cent of all the vitamins and minerals in a foodstuff, so you end up with empty calories. What are empty calories? They're calories which contain little in the way of nutrients – such as boiled sweets which are little more than sugar, water and flavourings. Alcohol has 'empty' calories too and, as I mentioned earlier, so have some commercially made desserts which are not really foods at all and which could not exist without the chemicals which bind them together. You must avoid these foods at all costs if you want to keep well hormonally.

Unrefined carbohydrates take a lot longer to digest so their sugars enter your bloodstream slowly, which is how your body likes its glucose. Refined carbohydrates, on the other hand, enter the bloodstream quickly, causing an instant insulin response. As I explained in the hormone section, the amount of insulin your body releases needs to be kept steady, and sudden glucose rushes due to eating refined carbohydrates is a wear on your body. This type of eating makes you tired and is what causes the binge-weight-gain cycle that makes you so miserable.

These are some examples of unrefined carbohydrates:

- potatoes
- peas
- sweetcorn
- untreated rice
- untreated pasta

- nuts and seeds such as sunflower, pumpkin, sesame
- vegetables
- lentils

## Refined carbohydrates: what's wrong with them?

The point is, we weren't designed to eat refined carbohydrates, any more than a dog is designed to eat cheese or a hedgehog to drink milk. We can put out milk for a hedgehog and it will drink it, and the dog will eat the cheese and they won't instantly be ill, but problems will come later when their internal organs just can't cope with the alien food. Much of our internal digestive workings are there to process fibrous foods, and if we eat a diet which has little in the way of fibre you're leaving these functions idle. Anybody who has suffered from diverticulitis which results from a refined diet will tell you how intensely painful it is, and it doesn't just go away. You also get the system 'backing-up' on itself with an unpleasant, sludgy residue left in your intestines.

Unrefined carbohydrates can cause mood swings, food cravings and binge eating – the reasons so many women feel their bodies are utterly chaotic in size, shape and consistency. They also cause water retention, stress and anxiety, and they don't help PMS, which is made a lot worse by the foods you tend to binge on, like crisps, cakes, chocolates and ready meals which are all highly refined and high in salt. In the process of refining carbohydrates, especially sugar and flour, present in most biscuits, cakes and breads, the mineral chromium is removed. Various studies confirm the ability of chromium to help you lose weight because it helps the body to lose fat and build muscle by increasing metabolic rate. Chromium is the central component in glucose tolerance.

Starch takes longer to digest than simple sugars so it provides a steady stream of energy, rather than the short 'blast' you get from unrefined sugars. However, the rate at which the starch in carbohydrates is released also varies, and, as I mentioned earlier, there is a measure of the relative increase in blood-sugar levels after eating similar amounts of different carbohydrate foods called the glycaemic index. Foods with a high glycaemic index bring rapid changes in blood-glucose levels. Low glycaemic index ratings result in glucose being released slowly, thus allowing your energy to last for longer.

Your central nervous system has an obligatory need for glucose, hence the need for chromium in the diet, and adults need 6g of glucose every hour, which is just 25 calories worth. The minimum glucose requirement for your brain is 70g a day, which comes to about 292 calories. You can tell how important it is to keep your glucose levels steady when you think of the dizziness and light-headedness you feel when you haven't eaten for a very long time and why, in severe cases of long-term dieting, the brain becomes affected and delusional. It is usually thought that the person concerned is simply getting eccentric, but in fact they are genuinely becoming incapable of thinking straight.

It is possible to contrive a diet consisting entirely of carbohydrate energy sources, fluids, vitamins and minerals. This would be fine for a short time but would lead eventually to muscle weakness and wasting because all the processes of renewal and growth in your body depend on proteins and fats as well as carbohydrates. The same thing applies to those elements of any diet. Of the many fashions in diet, the one currently doing the rounds is protein rich and carbohydrate free – again, a faddy diet which is doomed to failure. Why? Because human nature is such that unless you have a compelling medical, religious or conscientious reason for doing something, the incentive simply isn't there to keep it up for long. Eventually you are seduced by a round of toast, you're reminded of what you've been missing and you realize that the earth doesn't shift just because of your lapse. The faddy diet gets the elbow.

## How much you need

You should calculate your carbohydrate intakes thus:

Find your weight in kilograms e.g. 64kg (1kg=2.2lb)

If you are not very active, allow 3g carbohydrates per kg of weight = 192g a day

If you are moderately active, allow 4–5g per kg of weight = 256–320g a day

If you are active, allow 5–6g per kg of weight = 320–384g a day

For older people, high carbohydrate intakes can result in weight gain, so make sure that you don't go above 200g of carbohydrate per day.

These are only approximate figures. However, as you will see, the amounts of carbohydrates you should eat every day are much larger than the amount of fats or proteins, indicating that they must form the bulk of your daily diet for energy.

## Protein

Proteins are essential to form and maintain body tissues. All your processes of growth, maintenance and repair depend on protein. Most people eat enough protein or even too much, but they also have it at the wrong time of day, eating no protein for breakfast or lunch, then eating huge quantities in the evening. If you tend to eat just toast for breakfast and a salad for lunch, followed by meat with a sauce and maybe a pudding in the evening, you can send your protein levels rocketing.

Many bodybuilders display a strange gluttony when it comes to proteins, but surplus protein is not stored as muscle. The nitrogen is removed and excreted and the rest is either saved as energy in your muscles or stored as fat. It is not harmful to eat slightly excessive amounts of protein, but eventually you will gain weight as the extra calories will always be stored as fat.

## How much should I eat?

- You need about 0.75–1g of protein per kilogram of your body weight, per day.
- If you are very active, or if you are pregnant or breastfeeding, you will need 1–1.3g per kilogram per day.
- Sports people and bodybuilders could need up to 1.6g per kilogram per day.
- For example: if you are sixteen years old, weigh 50 kilos and are heavily into sport, you should eat between 50–60g of protein every day. If you are sixty years of age, weigh 62 kilos and are sedentary, you will need 46g of protein a day.
- You should try to balance out your meals by dividing your protein allowance into four, and trying to eat this amount at every meal.
- The ratio of carbohydrate to protein in any meal should be 2:1.

Protein and fats slow down the rate at which glucose is absorbed by the body, thus preventing that glucose 'rush' that can happen when a meal high in carbohydrates is eaten. In any event, at all stages of your life you need a sufficient amount of protein to keep going all the processes of maintenance and repair. A guide to the amounts in everyday foods are in the food file, page 294.

Look at this typical day's diet for twenty-two-year-old Caroline:

| | |
|---|---|
| Breakfast | Two cups coffee, apple. |
| On arriving at work | Two cups coffee. |
| 11.00 a.m. | Wholemeal salad sandwich, orange, coffee. |
| 1.00 p.m. | Salad of couscous with grilled vegetables, orange drink. |
| 7.00 p.m. | Pasta with chicken and tomato sauce, two slices garlic bread, side salad of green leaves, beetroot. Small portion apple pie with tablespoon single cream. Two glasses wine, coffee. |
| 9.30 p.m. | Two after-dinner mints, banana. |

What is wrong with this diet?

Caroline is not overweight, although she complains of 'monumental fatigue' which she puts down to the leftovers of a viral infection last year. She has brittle nails and is not happy with the condition of her hair, although she blames travelling on public transport in London and the level of pollution.

The real reason that Caroline feels tired and lacklustre is that her diet is entirely unbalanced. She starts the day badly with no breakfast, and although she eats a good salad sandwich during the morning and a healthy lunch, there is precious little in the way of protein, as she overdoses on more and more carbohydrates. It is rather like a 'toast overload', common to many an impoverished student. Toast and jam fills the gap, but provides little in the way of nutrients for the amount you are eating, plus you get that sugar low after an hour or so. Caroline's evening food consumption is also way too high with, by my reckoning, about 1,025 calories consumed in less than an hour. Her total calorie intake for the day is about 1,790, well within the correct range for her age group and maybe even a little low, but it is not providing her with the nutrients she needs for a full-time job, nor the protein which is essential for her looks. My recommendations would be to have a high-protein and carbohydrate breakfast such as boiled egg and wholemeal toast or muesli-based cereal and milk, oatcakes mid-morning with fruit, a lunch of fish salad with potatoes and a smaller evening meal of either fish or chicken with three cooked vegetables followed by fresh fruit salad.

So level out your protein intake! Have milk, bacon or an egg for breakfast, eat meat or cheese or nuts with lunch and have a smaller evening meal. In fact you won't need to try, because you won't feel like a big meal, I promise. The secret of your body weight and eating problems is regularity and balance. If your eating is out of control, your body will be out of control.

## Fats

I am not of the 'eat fat and you'll get fat' brigade. In my experience, people who avoid fats look dried out and dull. Banning cheese and butter is madness unless you really hate them – cheese is lovely for goodness sake! So how to manage a healthy eating plan without risking all for a ploughman's?

Excluding fat from your diet deprives your body of nutrients, as some vitamins cannot be absorbed without fat. You should have in total about 70g of fat in your daily diet, of which about 21.5g may be saturated animal fat. You need to eat about 25mg of fat a day to help you absorb vitamins A, D, E and K, and also betacarotene which your body can convert into vitamin A. Omega 6 fatty acids are needed to help produce hormone-like substances which help control many functions including inflammation and blood flow. An adult needs very little – about 4g a day, which is about a couple of teaspoons of sunflower oil, or a handful of almonds. Omega 3 fatty acids are needed in tiny amounts but they are still essential to help your blood clot and reduce inflammation, and you can get enough from a handful of nuts or a small serving of oily fish like mackerel. Many people who suffer from arthritis and skin problems find oily fish or fish oils to be beneficial.

## Saturated fats

The real baddies in the fat camp are saturated fats – the ones which lodge in your arteries if you're not careful or take no exercise. Saturated fats come from animal products, so while I recommend you don't become paranoid about cheese, meat and butter, just watch the amount you eat. I never look at total fat contents on labels because I know I need the good fats from vegetables, seeds and nuts, but my eye lands straight on the amount of saturated fat. The daily limit for a woman is 21.5g, so tot up your intake from that. It's frighteningly easy to consume more than a whole day's allowance in one plateful of food, but don't panic just yet. We all have holidays when we eat way over the amount we should, and weddings and parties and all manner of occasions when we go over the top. Just don't make it too often. Life might not be worth living without a few treats, but at least you've got a life. I think a life with a few restrictions, a bit of order and control and a superb body is better than not having one at all, don't you?

Here are some examples of the total fat and saturated fat contents of everyday foods, which I have given you to show how easy it is to 'overspend' your fat allowance! See how one full cooked breakfast uses an entire day's allowance, while white fish may be eaten in quantity. For full information on fats in your diet, look at food labels and start counting!

| Food | Total Fat (g) | Saturated Fat (g) |
| --- | --- | --- |
| All Bran cereal, 30g | 1.5 | 0.2 |
| Alpen, 30g | 3.3 | 0.6 |
| Apple | trace | trace |
| Avocado pear, half | 14.6 | 3.0 |
| Bacon and egg, average portion | 29.0 | 10.0 |
| Banana | 0.3 | 0.1 |
| Beef stir-fry, average portion | 31.0 | 10.0 |
| Bubble and squeak, fried, average portion | 18.2 | 9.6 |
| Cheesecake, slice | 43.0 | 23.0 |
| Chicken breast, 150g | 4.0 | 1.0 |
| Chicken nuggets, 6 | 13.0 | 3.0 |
| Chips from burger bar, 150g | 17.0 | 6.4 |
| Cod, baked, 150g | 1.4 | 0.4 |
| Cooked breakfast, full English | 72.0 | 28.0 |

| Food | Total Fat (g) | Saturated Fat (g) |
|------|---------------|-------------------|
| Croissant with butter and jam | 20.0 | 5.0 |
| Danish pastry | 19.0 | 6.0 |
| Egg, boiled | 5.4 | 1.5 |
| Egg, scrambled, on toast | 45.0 | 20.0 |
| Fillet steak, 150g | 16.0 | 7.0 |
| Milk, full-fat, 250ml | 11.0 | 7.0 |
| Milk, skimmed, 250ml | 0.3 | 0.3 |
| Muesli, 30g, and milk, 150ml | 7.0 | 2.0 |
| Pot Noodles | 9.0 | not known |
| Rasher bacon | 5.0 | 2.0 |
| Salmon steak, fresh, 150g | 13.0 | 2.0 |
| Spaghetti in tomato sauce, 150g | 0.8 | 0.2 |
| Sponge cake, 1 slice | 18.0 | 6.0 |
| Tuna fish, fresh, portion, 100g | 8.0 | 1.4 |
| Vegetable curry, average portion | 15.0 | 3.0 |
| Waldorf salad, 150g tub | 79.0 | 11.0 |
| White bread, large slice | 0.5 | 0.1 |
| Wholemeal bread, slice | 0.7 | 0.1 |

Top choices: wholemeal bread; chicken; fish; skimmed milk; fruit and vegetables.

## Vitamins and Minerals

The most important rule for starting a good eating plan is to think 'nutrient dense'. You know that you need a balance of all the vitamins and minerals, plus the correct amounts of carbohydrates, fats and proteins, but many people eat a lot of food which is nutrient poor, good examples being biscuits, sweets or very low-calorie products. The reason why these can be low in nutrients is what I call 'spinning out' or 'blowing up' the ingredients. Reducing the nutrient value of a sauce to practically nothing by adding water and flavourings is one manufacturer's ploy, another is expanding a product with air so you actually get less than half the product once the air is removed. This is very bad in my view, and it is much more satisfying to eat a smaller portion of the real thing. It is easy to eat nutrient dense as long as you know which foods are the powerhouses. For the examples below, I have given some ridiculous amounts of food to illustrate just how you can be barking up the wrong tree when it comes to which food is rich in a certain vitamin.

## Vitamin A

What it does for you:

- Helps form photosensitive pigment in the eyes
- Helps maintain healthy skin, and prevent acne
- A powerful antioxidant vitamin
- Essential for healthy cell turnover

You should have 600mcg a day. You can find this amount in:

- 200 apples
- 85 tablespoons sweetcorn
- 15 small pots of plain yoghurt
- 1 portion spinach
- one Spanish omelette – with 2 eggs, red and yellow pepper, onions, mushrooms and few small potatoes, sliced
- but just 85g carrots!

## Vitamin C

What it does for you:

- Maintains healthy connective tissue, gums and skin

You should have about 40mg a day. You can find this amount in:

- 5 portions peas
- 7 apples
- one Spanish omelette
- half an orange
- but just a quarter of a red pepper!

## Vitamin E

What it does for you:

- An essential anti-oxidant

You should have 6mg a day. You can find this amount in:

- 25 jacket potatoes
- 4 bowls All Bran
- 2 fillets salmon
- 20 hazelnuts
- 10 almonds
- 1 avocado
- 1 tbsp sunflower seeds
- but just one teaspoon of wheatgerm oil!

## Vitamin B complex

These are a group of vitamins which work together, including:

- thiamine (B1) You need 0.8mg a day
- riboflavin (B2). You need 1.1mg a day
- niacin (B3). You need 13mg a day
- pyridoxine (B6). You need 1.2mg a day
- pantothenic acid (B5). You need 3–7mg a day
- folic acid. You need 200mcg a day
- B12. You need 1.2mcg a day

What it does for you:

- Improves your mental attitude

- Helps fight air and seasickness
- Keeps the nervous system functioning

## Foods high in vitamin B:

- eggs
- pork
- milk
- steak
- lentils
- leeks
- but top marks go to lamb's liver

## Iron

## What it does for you:

- Carries oxygen in the blood to all tissues
- Alleviates tiredness and lethargy

## You need 10–18mg every day. You can find this amount in:

- 10 bowls of porridge
- 1½ bowls Special K
- 12 sardines
- 5 portions baked beans
- 10 bags of peanuts
- 100 small pots of plain yoghurt
- but just one chicken vindaloo (or other curry) – the curry powder is the high source of iron here!

## Calcium

## What it does for you:

- Vital to the development and maintenance of the skeleton
- Plays a vital role in the smooth contraction of muscle
- Important in regulating all metabolic processes

You need about 700mg per day. You can find this amount in:

- 87 cream crackers
- 29 bowls of All Bran
- 2 portions vegetable lasagne
- 2 cheese and tomato pizzas
- 2 bowls Ready Brek
- 2 portions macaroni cheese
- 3 portions chicken korma
- 2 slices cheese and egg quiche
- 56g Cheddar cheese
- half a litre of any milk
- 3 pots yoghurt
- but only six sardines!

## What's best to eat

So – if you can only limit your meals to a small choice, here are the very best for nutrient density:

- fillet steak, jacket potato, pepper salad
- Spanish omelette with salad dressed with a wheatgerm oil and vinegar dressing
- lamb's liver with onions and vegetables, fruit salad with custard made from 250ml skimmed milk
- roast, skinless chicken or pork with carrots and potatoes
- Brussels sprouts and cheese soufflé
- grilled sardines on toast

This has been a general overview of the type of food you need to eat to keep in the best health and the best shape. Overall, it is also a good way to eat for your hormonal health. The diet section (page 185) gives you the complete picture about eating for specific problems such as stress, anxiety, pregnancy or the menopause, but I hope you see from this last section that the most important element of your diet is balance. Here are other things to remember:

- Drink a lot of water.
- Eat the required amount of carbohydrate for every kilo you weigh (see above).
- Don't wait until the evening for your first burst of protein: you must always have some with breakfast.
- Don't be fat phobic – the fats in nuts, seeds and oils are good for you.

# The Way to Lose Weight

Most of us want to lose weight. Although this book is about hormones, it's obviously more about your weight. But which way to lose weight – count fat grams, carbohydrate units, calories? The next section should answer this most important question.

## Do Calories Count?

The role and importance of the calorie is still misunderstood, especially by people who want to lose weight. They will often feel that all calories are bad, that they must somehow have as few as possible and burn off the ones they do eat. Considering that between the time you go to sleep at night and wake up in the morning, you'll have burned around a calorie a minute – 480 in all – you'll realize that your biggest calorie expenditure is in being alive! An obsessive preoccupation with calories is not only bad for you, it's ineffective. Let Paula, who describes herself as 'a serial yo-yo dieter' tell you her story:

I'm looking at a photograph of myself taken about thirteen years ago, just after I'd spent a year losing 25 kilos (four stone). I was very slim. Six months later, I'd piled the whole lot back on. The trouble was that I was always too impatient about losing my weight. I knew people who had lost weight on 1,000 calories a day and it became a kind of competition. It seemed to take so long, so I thought I could go one better by eating only 800 calories, and then 500. I even tried to beat that as well!

The problem was, I felt so terrible. I always had a cold or sore throat, because I was eating so little. I had nothing for breakfast, maybe an apple for lunch and when I got home I'd eat two tins of tomatoes on one slice of toast with loads of salt. I don't know what it was about the salt, but I craved it. Sometimes I had some milk in tea, but it felt like pure fat. Obviously I didn't eat anything like 500 calories, so on the days when I ate 400 or even 350 calories I'd write in my diary, 'I made it!!' If I went as high as 500 calories, I felt a failure.

It never occurred to me that my body needed feeding for reasons other than simply getting from A to B. My hair looked bad because it wasn't getting any nourishment. I was tired because my muscles had no energy stores, but I thought I had enough fat to live on!

I simply thought that all calories were bad, and of course the end of each diet meant the start of several months of eating everything in sight.

This then is the big calorie misunderstanding. It is good to have an awareness of calories, because it's lack of awareness of exactly what calories are and their purpose that leads people to a poor diet and an imbalance of nutrients. Why? Because you might think that eating 1,200 calories a day was all that mattered but, of course, you can eat 1,200 calories a day in Mars bars. So it isn't just the calories you eat, but where they come from that's important. Then there's the element of competition – that somehow you've succeeded if you can eat less. As Paula said when describing her starvation diet to me, calorie allowances set a level which once overshot indicates failure. Many people eat slightly too many calories and binge without restraint as a result. Eating too few calories works in the opposite way, engendering a feeling of success and jubilation when in fact the individual is doing herself no favours.

So what are calories, why do you need them and do they make you fat? Here are some calorie facts:

- Calories give you energy, and energy gives you the ability to work.
- Energy keeps you alive.
- Calories make muscle movement possible.
- Calories supply extra needs when growing, in pregnancy and when breastfeeding.
- After eating, your body makes extra heat and more energy is needed to cover this which is why eating raises your metabolic rate and burns more calories.
- You actually burn more calories in twenty-four hours doing nothing at all. At one calorie a minute even when sleeping, that's 1,440 calories a day used in inactivity.
- Calories don't make you fat – it's how you use them which determines whether you will lay down fat.

Choice of calories matters. For example, ten small KitKats have only 1,100 calories and although you'd get thin on them, you'd be pretty unhealthy. Food which has a lot of calories in a small amount, such as fats like cheese and butter, or foods with both fat and sugar, such as rich fruit cake, are called 'energy dense'. Food which is energy dense has a valuable purpose. For example, if you were an Arctic explorer or a foot soldier about to trek fifty miles across an inhospitable landscape with a pack on your back, you would not want to be coping with a heavy, full stomach from 1,000 calories worth of meat and two veg followed by a large fruit salad and yoghurt. In some situations you need a lot of energy packed into the smallest possible amount, so the 1,200 calories from two small pieces of fruit cake would be the perfect solution. On the other hand, if you have a sedentary job and go home to a lively toddler or house full of adolescents, you are using fewer calories for physical exercise while needing to stay on top form mentally, so you would be looking at nutrient-dense, low-calorie foods which would provide enough carbohydrates to keep your energy levels steady. Steady energy comes from food with a low glycaemic index, and there is a list of these foods on page 304.

So, here are some examples of foods which are high in nutrients and low in calories (about 250 calories) for the quantity you are eating and other foods or meals which provide the same calories with a lot less goodness in them:

| High nutrient/low calorie | High calorie/low nutrient |
| --- | --- |
| 40g roasted peanuts | 500ml strong cider |
| 2 boiled eggs and 1 slice toast | 6 after-dinner mints |
| 1 banana, 2 apples, 20 grapes | 95g slice pepperoni pizza |
| chicken breast, broccoli, carrots, gravy | 1 chicken quarter-pounder |
| | 1 battered fish portion |
| | 1 individual apple pie |

I'm sure you can see where I'm heading. When calculating an ideal weight-loss or weight-maintenance diet you need to consider not just the calories, but where they're coming from. The chicken and vegetable meal is high in nutrients because it has protein, vitamins, minerals, carbohydrates and a little fat. The fruit option has one of the best ingredients – water – as well as the staying power of the banana and the lasting carbohydrate content of the apples and grapes, and the boiled egg and toast contains proteins, B vitamins and fibre.

But how does the average person know what is in their food? Well, my section on nutrition sets the ball rolling, and of course not even I as a nutritionist know precisely every vitamin and trace mineral content of a given meal. What I do think is important though, is that you have a working knowledge of what food contains because, coming back to hormones, the efficient working of most of our hormone systems depend on the right balance of natural chemicals in our bodies, sugar being the most obvious one. If you consistently choose food from the 'not so good' list, you might be restricting calories by eating small amounts, but your levels of sugar and fat will be high – resulting in the inevitable low moods, lethargy and irritability.

A major benefit of proper meals which have bulk without the calories, is that they take time to eat. Going back to my piece of fruit cake, how long would it take you to eat a slice? Three minutes? Less than that? Yet a largish slice would pack a hefty 600–800 calories, and you'd probably still be prowling around for something else. A full roast lunch with chicken and potatoes could have half the calories, and take fifteen minutes to put away. So why does this matter? Because it takes your body time to register the 'full' signal in your brain, and eating hurriedly generally means that you eat a lot more food. As any woman keen on her diet and figure will tell you, grabbing a snack is the quickest way to load calories on board without even remembering that you ate them. Having said that, you can hardly roast a chicken or boil eggs while sitting in your office or travelling on the tube, so the fresh fruit or even the peanut option are other good choices. This is what I mean by 'which calories'? It's up to you and your lifestyle, but be aware of what you're getting, and don't be calorie-phobic like Paula.

## Dying to be Slim – When Dieting Turns Ugly

### Anorexia Nervosa

The word 'anorexia' actually means loss of appetite, and mustn't be confused with anorexia nervosa. Loss of appetite happens when people are ill or have had operations and have lost their appetite because they don't feel well. Anorexia nervosa is depression of your appetite which is brought on consciously. You don't want to eat, you won't eat, and gradually your appetite diminishes. Even if it doesn't diminish, your determination not to eat is usually too strong to allow the food to win.

Anorexia nervosa sufferers are below the normal range of weight for their age and height by about 15 per cent. This amount of fat loss leads to hormonal disturbances, and when three consecutive periods have failed to appear, it is a sign that menstruation has stopped.

Eating disorders are not primarily about food. They are about psychological turmoil and underlying distress, and the range of treatments include cognitive behavioural therapy anxiety management, nutritional management and family counselling. It is not within the scope of this book to address the issue of serious eating disorders. However, the teens are a time of intense interest in your body, and the more common fixation is of being fat, or having disproportionate legs, bottom or stomach. When your cycles are establishing themselves and your body shape is changing rapidly, you can look in the mirror almost every day and see something different about yourself. It is important that you take an interest in your body, learn how to look after it and make it as healthy and attractive as you possibly can – I receive far too many letters from girls who insist that every feature of their bodies repulses them – but your best bet is to exercise and watch your diet, not cut back on nutrients. Eating very little never works in the long run because nature takes over and forces you to eat by making food your central obsession. Food doesn't make you fat. Food is fuel and, if anything, it makes you beautiful. Beauty is the entire effect, and a glowing skin, strong nails and glossy hair are even more important for attracting a mate than your figure.

Here are just six of many amazing things your body does in the course of a week:

- Your heart beats more than 700,000 times.
- You breathe over 121,000 times.
- Your stomach produces nearly a gallon of digestive juices.
- Your entire outer skin cells are replaced.
- Your hair grows two millimetres.
- 1,750 gallons of blood passes through your kidneys.

You can't do all this if you hardly eat!

I don't think that if you have an intense fear of food and getting fat, that the emphasis should be on weight gain. Going from starvation to health shouldn't start with a calorie jump of 2,000 a day – in my opinion. I think it is far too threatening, and the steps should be gradual. The emphasis on food should be replaced by something else, with meals being restricted at first to a little milk and some vegetables and fruit. It is particularly important for you to know that you are in no way abnormal in being afraid of getting fat, in fact a large percentage of the population feels exactly as you do, but perhaps do not go to such extremes. These first few steps can often be highly successful because they introduce glucose to your brain, and when glucose is lacking it affects clear thinking and brings on depression. Start by raising glucose levels with milk and sugar, and you might then find it easier to be positive about the future.

## Bulimia Nervosa

Another severe form of body chaos is bulimia nervosa. Like anorexia nervosa, it is a psychological condition which is brought on by the woman herself, as opposed to vomiting through illness. The difference between the two disorders is that sufferers of bulimia seem to be keen to talk about it and even, as we know from several high-profile cases, discuss it openly in front of millions of strangers. I have had a lot of contact with bulimics, and I know one thing for certain: it is not a disorder where people only stuff themselves to the hilt, gorging on bagfuls of strange, unpalatable food, I have known countless women who hold down good jobs and positions of authority who will eat a normal lunch and carefully bring back exactly half of it – and this is their way of life. On the face of it this is not as chaotic as eating the tons of food scenario, and it could even be said to be ordered and calculated, and it goes on in just about every ladies' loo in every corporate building and every restaurant in the land. People tell me about it in the same way they would describe going to the hairdresser or for a manicure, and for them it is a reasonable course of action to prevent something they don't want.

I have had a few clients who have wanted to conquer this compulsion, and for a while they stick carefully to the structured diet that I give them, which always results in stable weight and better energy levels, but it rarely lasts. Why go to all the trouble of being careful when you can eat anything and then vomit? The 'I want it yesterday' mentality is the downfall of many women, and if you haven't the patience, you'll never do it. It is not normal to vomit your food wilfully. For such women who would pride themselves on being ordered, in control and at the peak of their powers, I would say that this habit – and it is no more than a grotesque habit after all – is proof that they are not all that they would wish to be thought. I have little time for bulimics of this calibre, and especially those who return somebody's hospitality by being sick. If ever there were a case for etiquette guidance, it would be, 'never vomit in your hostess's bathroom'.

## How Anorexia Nervosa and Bulimia Cause Chaos

In anorexia and bulimia, a proportion of sufferers have delayed gastric emptying. Your internal digestive process operates on a system of constant 'throughput'. In a healthy person, digestion should be uncomplicated, should cause no irritation and should run smoothly. As Consultant Gastro-enterologist Dr Roger Chapman told me, 'There is no value at all in fasting, and people who have prolonged periods of not eating, such as in crash dieting, can have harmful conditions arise such as bile sludge and gallstones. This "sludge" is simply food which isn't being pushed along because your digestion is grinding to a halt. Remember that your digestive system is there for a purpose, and leaving it to lie idle does no good at all.'

## The Miracle of Homeostasis and Leptin

I wanted to end this section on a cheering note, and you can't get more cheering than the miracle of homeostasis. Why is it cheering? Because it can mean that whatever weight gains you've made, you can return to a normal size much more easily than you think. This doesn't mean that you don't have to do any hard work – would that I could promise you that! – but it means that it is easier than you think to return to normal, even if you have been fat for decades.

Let me explain. Homeostasis is defined as the maintenance of a constant physical or chemical state. Many processes in your body are under homeostatic control, which is similar to the process of a thermostat, where temperature is brought back to a certain point according to where the thermostat is set. In fact, your temperature regulation is a good example of homeostatic control. The set point for body temperature is 37 C. If your temperature goes above this point you'll start sweating to cool down your outer skin surface. If your temperature goes too low you'll shiver, and your basal metabolic rate increases to bring your core temperature back up to where it should be. There are other functions in which homeostats plays a part, such as when insulin is triggered to respond to a sudden rise in your blood-sugar levels. Sodium and potassium also regulate each other. So you have these continual processes responding to each other and sitting like animals on guard, ready to spring into action if our lives are threatened by a deviation from the set point.

The set-point theory suggests that your weight is kept constant by similar homeostasis. If this theory is correct, we all have a set level of body fat, and changes in weight trigger a mechanism to bring our weight back to this point.

There is also a theory about a mechanism known as an 'adipostat', which keeps your levels of fat constant in spite of wide deviations in your physical activity or fat intake. There are several theories about the adipostat which are not proven, but the protein leptin, a Greek word meaning 'thinness', has been widely investigated and studied in recent years and is known to play a large part in detecting the state of the individual's fat stores.

While size might not be genetically pre-determined, fat children with a poor parental example can find their appetites difficult to control as they grow up. Why do some people lose weight only to pile it back on again? Is it purely down to lack of willpower? Surely, if it were just a matter of determination, these women would succeed? After all, all the health-club memberships and treatments, the expenditure on books, magazines, diets, videos and health farms point to someone taking the whole process very seriously indeed. So what goes wrong? With so much at stake, how come a simple thing like food and appetite gets the better of them time and again?

You are born with a certain number of fat cells. Between the ages of six and seven you have a sudden increase in the number of these cells and another burst at puberty. Girls go on producing fat cells longer than boys because they need them for reproduction, but if a child has been overfed he or she will have a greater number of cells. Your brain is constantly monitoring the size of your fat cells because they are a major factor in survival. Leptin is a protein which is released from your fat cells at night. Its job is to tell your brain how your fat stores are faring by sending signals to your hypothalamus, the detector of the piece.

The hypothalamus is a gland situated just below your brain. It is like a thermostat, sensitively monitoring the overall state of play between your pituitary gland, ovaries and uterus and, indeed, these hormones constantly respond to each other. Receptors in the hypothalamus see how much leptin is in your blood, and when the amount of leptin signals that your fat stores are well stocked it stops your drive to eat. If you have a lot of fat cells, your drive to eat won't stop until they are all stocked, so production of leptin continues and you want to go on eating. Food is more appealing and your sense of taste is heightened as your body encourages you to keep eating, and this might be why – a big 'might' as it is still just a theory – some people get an overwhelming fancy to certain foods even when their stomachs are full. Leptin is a new story, and it is a story that is only just being understood. It might explain, however, why people who only become fat after adolescence can lose the weight more easily than someone who has been fat since childhood, although it is still linked to childhood feeding rather than genetics. You mustn't think, though, that if you were a fat child you are somehow doomed. Training your appetite levels might be more of a challenge but people do it successfully all the time.

Other experts disagree with the whole leptin story, even though there is no dispute that leptin exists. They say that the set-point theory is purely psychological, arising from your personal tastes in clothes, your measurements and so on. What they maintain happens is that you strive to achieve a result by adopting habits you don't enjoy, such as exercising a particular way, eating foods you have to force down at times which don't suit you, and it is these changes in habit rather than a problem with food, fat cells or leptin, which cause you to give up dieting. I feel that most people can change habits if there's enough at stake and if long enough is allowed – rather like my 'changing your territory' advice, but you really have to give it a fair chance to establish itself. Whichever is the true cause of weight and appetite problems, you end up helplessly concluding that it is genetically inevitable – the 'I was born a fat person' theory.

Deviations in weight which don't affect homeostasis are the run-of-the-mill causes we all experience from time to time: the couple of stressful days when we don't eat, the tummy bug or flu virus, the heavy weekend of celebrations when we eat and drink enough for an army – these are recognized by your body as small 'blips' on your normally steady graph, and while you might complain of a tight waistband, a few extra kilos or even a weight loss – the changes are insignificant and temporary.

The major deviations happen when you crash diet. A period of several weeks without the usual calories, a sustained increase in exercise or a marked difference in the type of food eaten such as going from a normal diet to a protein-only regime, all cause a shock to your system which makes your metabolism slam on the brakes. No more calories coming in? Save the ones you've got. This is why metabolic rates are always decreased by long-term decreases in calories, although your metabolism is rarely, if ever, 'messed up' by dieting, even if it is as severe as anorexia nervosa or bulimia. You'll be glad to know that in even the worst of cases, metabolism soon returns to normal when a stable routine is established again. This doesn't mean that you necessarily go back to being fat again, you need to understand the difference between your metabolic rate and the effect of calories. If your metabolic rate returns to normal after being slowed by too few calories, as long as you maintain an energy balance between calories eaten and calories used in activity, your weight will remain stable.

I believe that there is a set point for all of us. For years a friend of mine called Amanda tried to keep her weight below 48 kilos by severe dieting, eating only about 800 calories a day. When she relaxed and ate only 1,200 calories a day, her weight went up to 51 kilos. She continually pushed it back down to 48 kilos because she professed to feeling better at that weight, but always it rose back up to 51 kilos. Now how can this be, you might think, when you have to eat 3,500 calories a day to gain even half a kilo and she had gained 3 kilos? I like to think that her body was happier at 51 kilos, and this was confirmed when she decided to give in and give up the dieting. She assumed that her weight would rise inexorably to about 63 kilos, but it didn't. She remained at 51 kilos for the next eighteen years, neither rising above nor dipping below that magic number. I can only assume that in all the years she tried to be a lower weight, her body simply didn't want to do it through some pre-determined homeostat, and I have been a firm believer in the set-point theory ever since. Moreover, I have seen how successful people can be the minute they apply a measure of routine and restriction to their lives.

So if we have a pre-determined level of fat stores, how come anyone ever manages to lose weight and keep it off? Surely we'd go straight back to our original level of fat stores the minute we eat normally again? Well, that depends on what you call 'normally'. If someone weighs 32 kilos more than they should, they can't have been eating normally. If they weigh less than 6 kilos more than usual, they are probably eating normally but not being very active or careful. If it's as simple as a few hundred extra calories a week, and you've been slim for many years beforehand, the weight will drop off and stay off as your body gratefully returns to its set point. You haven't been allowing it to return by sheer weight of extra calories on a consistent basis, but a small reduction will do the trick as long as it is maintained. You must also keep pace with inevitable changes in metabolism that come with age, so as your clock begins to set itself ever so slightly slower you need to be aware of this and adjust yourself accordingly. Age-related changes in calorie needs amount only to about 200 a day, but not acknowledging this can result in 5.5 kilos of weight gain in a year. In the section on exercise I'll be exploring the question of metabolism control through weight training, so don't despair just yet!

You can reset your programme, but you should make sure you start by banishing fluctuations in your routine. Here are some reasons for the fluctuations:

- Trying to maintain too low a weight.
  As in Amanda's story, you need to be aware of just how far you can push your body. If your weight always creeps back up to a level point you might just be asking too much of it if you are constantly striving to lose more weight than that. Try to heed what your body is telling you!

- Trying to stick to an unrealistic regime.
  Female bodybuilders spend many weeks during their training season eating

a bizarre diet to maintain low body fat. Jockeys also embark on extremely low calorie and fluid intakes to reduce their weight for competition. Needless to say, the minute a normal and varied diet is consumed again off-season, their weight will rise because the body gratefully retains water again. Sodium is severely restricted on a bodybuilder's diet, and this means that water will be lost from the body at a faster rate – when sodium is reintroduced, water will be retained more quickly as the body gratefully re-hydrates! This is unlikely to be fat-weight, but the scales still register an increase.

- Too much variation in the amounts you eat.
  Eating a lot one day and very little the next, eating huge meals sometimes and picking at other times – this results in weight fluctuations of as much as 4.5kg either way. This usually has no sinister consequences for your health, although it is now thought that certain conditions like heart disease later in life are linked to 'yo-yo dieting'. Certainly from my own experience, if you eat in this chaotic way you can get depressed and irritable, particularly if the fluctuations are self-imposed in order to control hunger pangs. Here again, hormones come into the picture because you have already learned about adrenalin stimulation when you are particularly hungry, and progesterone levels rising after a meal. It is never a good idea to be this chaotic. Some experts argue that ancient man ate chaotically because he had to eat a lot when food was plentiful and go hungry at other times, but there is a lot about ancient man that wouldn't work for us today. They didn't live long, either!

- A cycle of eat and starve can only be broken by a psychological commitment to routine – there are no short cuts!

- The energy balance being out of line.
  People often ask me how much they should be eating and what their ideal weight should be. I tell them they will get their answers by looking in the mirror. What do you look like? Do you look tired and puffy? Overweight or underweight? The answer is that if you are 19kg overweight, whatever you are eating, it is more than you need.

- There are no set limits for your number of calories, and say you were using up in excess of 3,000 calories a day, you could eat 3,000 calories and not gain a gram. The other side of the coin is that even if you only eat 1,500 calories a day but you only use up 1,400 calories, you will steadily store fat. This happens, unfortunately, when people are confined to wheelchairs, or have illnesses which restrict activity. Low energy levels don't mean you'll automatically get fat, but you would need to balance that energy, and good ways to do this would be to eat meals which are nutrient dense but low calorie, like salads or fruit mousses. This way you get a nice plateful of food which is appetizing, without the calorie load.

## Your Body – Giving It the Final Word

As you will have guessed, I am a great believer in the body almost as a personality in its own right. You are told to 'listen to your body', but it is something most of us rarely do. It means being aware that your body has only one way of telling you what it needs, what it can do without and what it really hates. If you are currently having a nightmare with your weight, remember that good old homeostasis will restore the status quo speedily if you let it, so your panic and depression about your size are not really justified. Nobody needs to be fat. You are no different from anybody else. You get back on track much more easily than you thought possible by having faith and adopting reasonable eating habits. In the next section I am going to give you several diet plans to help you with your moods or weight gain, so cheer up! Your body chaos is soon to be a thing of the past.

# Beat Your **Body Chaos**

In the first half of this book, I looked at body chaos as you would recognize it. Now I have some solutions for you, from a superb weight-loss diet, to individual plans for special hormonal needs. You *can* overcome your body chaos, and you will.

# Chapter Seven

# Mental Attitude

Body chaos, as you have seen, is a huge topic. Your hormones drive your emotions, moods and ultimately your every waking moment, but I couldn't write about your body without also talking about your mind. Remember, this is your mind and my mind as well, because as a woman I have experienced most of what I have written about so far. I also know that the biggest hurdle is your mind. Rather as we women are never really convinced that our bottom doesn't look big in an item of clothing, it's hard to accept that body chaos is ever going to end. Most of it boils down to your mental attitude, and if there's anything that I've learnt through researching this book, it's that women who profess to suffer no hormone problems, usually have positive, busy lives which suit their temperaments. There are no hard and fast rules about being busy or fulfilled: if you are a quiet, reclusive type, you won't be happy in a laughing crowd of friends; if you can't stand your own company and tend to brood, your headaches and pains will feel worse when you're cooped up on a wet weekend in February. So don't forget to find a way of life which suits your temperament, otherwise you'll suffer from one of the worst body chaos symptoms: stress.

The key to overcoming your body chaos is your mental attitude. You need to keep to a routine, discipline and self-respect. This might sound rather pompous, but it's not meant to be. For the past few years we've been bombarded with images of 'girl power' and women's rights, and this is no more than that kind of mind set. I well remember the days when women didn't stand up for themselves and were treated as second-rate citizens, and I think that also went for the attitudes of doctors towards our hormonal and weight problems. It was your GP who gave out diet sheets, your GP who told you that there was no point in hoping for a flat stomach when you'd had a baby. Mercifully those days have long gone, so my mantra of routine, discipline and self-respect is no more than an acknowledgement of how far we have come. If you want to feel and look better, *go for it*!

While you need no more than a sense of purpose, perspective and vision in order to get you going, it is easier said than done. With most of us doing jobs we hate just for the salary cheque, living with people we can't stand for the sake of others, or having to embrace responsibilities that drain us of time and mental energy, isn't it a mite unrealistic to expect us to channel any reserves into planning our lives better? Well, no, it's not. If your life is so dull, boring or empty, couldn't it be that you're doing something wrong? Other people manage to be happy and calm and content, so what's their secret? I once gave up smoking successfully after many years of failed attempts simply by asking myself what non-smokers did when they stopped for a coffee or came to the end of a meal. If I sat there expecting a cigarette, what were they expecting? If I had no trouble declining a slice of corned beef or salami when it was offered to me, how come I struggled when the biscuits did the rounds? It was only by looking at these thought processes and turning them on their heads that I got any answers. Non-smokers didn't struggle because cigarettes meant absolutely nothing to them. I didn't struggle with the corned beef and salami because I was similarly indifferent. All right, so if it was as easy as pretending you don't like cream cakes we'd all be happy, but you take my point. There's no magic cure, so it might be worth cultivating a few tricks. Put washing-up liquid in the dinner leftovers if you're tempted to finish them up, get some chickens so you can throw the second half of your lunch out to them with a clear conscience. Whatever works for you, do it.

If you have a weight problem and it's dominating your life and you say you've tried everything, are you sure that's true? Many people tell me this, but when I ask them what exactly they've tried it usually turns out that they've been on a couple of diets for a month, exercised for a few weeks and tried a few slimmers' biscuits. When nothing happened – meaning that the results they expected didn't materialize – they gave up, thereby guaranteeing that nothing would happen! Yes, I can understand it. If you're not having a good time eating healthy food and denying yourself the goodies you like, you might as well not have a good time and eat everything you do like. As I see it, this is unsuccessful living. It means you're expecting to have a rotten time, you're expecting failure and misery, you're permanently dis-appointed with yourself and there's nothing you can do about it. But you must take control and conquer this weakness – this lack of energy that somehow you know how to help yourself – but you can't be bothered. The solution can't be dialled up like a pizza. Nobody can eat properly for you or exercise on your behalf. You must exercise some discipline simply because otherwise, nothing gets done.

So take control! It sounds as if you'll be putting aside the concerns of your children, parents or career but you won't. Simply decide what you want to eat, when you want to exercise and rather than try to fit it in, make a schedule which includes these needs. No, it's not just about 'having a bit of time for me' because that can mean anything: it's about sorting out what you do want, and discarding the wrapping.

# The Benefits of Routine

## It Cuts Down On Stress

You might believe that an open-ended life is the best one for you: eating when you feel hungry, eating whatever food comes to hand, staying at work until late or taking work home with you – these are not the signs of an organized person and indeed, they suggest that you are insecure about your work. You will insist that it isn't work, that it is pure pleasure, but this is rarely true. You will be worrying about how much work the next person is getting done, how they are scaling the ladder in your absence. This leads to negative stress.

## It Helps Others

It actually helps others if your routine becomes part of their routine. I have hours when I'm in and hours when I'm out, and knowing my availability saves others stress too. If you think you can reach somebody on their mobile phone any time of the day or night you can make ten calls and leave ten messages and still not have a clue about whether the person has received them, or even if they're in the country! Set aside certain hours for yourself, stick with them and do the same for your meals. Eating at set times also spares uncertainty, and believe me, nobody ever lost their job or the respect of others simply because they went for lunch. Think you can't stop a meeting at a precise time and ask for lunch? My son is a diabetic and asks for this consideration all the time. Nobody ever objects.

## It Limits Choices, Saves Money and Time

This is really the same as saving stress. If you go into a supermarket without a clear idea of what you're going to buy, you've got a dazzling array of about 1,000 potential meals to choose from – a time-consuming choice. By planning and devoting a day to each meal, you have the problem completely sewn up.

## It Stops Snacking

Some diet programmes downplay the reasons why you eat. Some might even tell you that there is nothing good about eating and that dieting is a piece of cake. Well, this isn't my approach. Eating is rewarding and nice, otherwise you wouldn't be doing it. However, I believe that if you know what holds you back from dieting and what attracts you to food you will be able to confront this habit and handle it. Eating isn't like smoking. You can decide never to have a cigarette in the house again but you can't do that with food. But instead of food taking its rightful place in your life as planned meal stops, you eat food you don't even remember having. You get engrossed in a film and suddenly look at the coffee table to see an empty crisp packet, wine glass and apple core. We tend to eat in the same places, with the same people and at the same times, whether or not we're hungry or even aware of what we're doing. A coffee? Out comes the biscuit tin. Stop off for a cooling lager? Have a packet of peanuts as well. Having set mealtimes is one thing because we all have to eat, but fitting in food to an empty timetable when you aren't hungry is something else. As with all the advice in this book, having snacks is fine in itself if you have no physical problems, but if you are struggling to lose weight these are the areas you might want to address.

# All In the Mind

If you are ever going to conquer your body chaos, you have to start with the chaos which is raging in your mind. Here are the prime culprits:

- Lack of willpower – you have the will but it has no direction and no power.
- Lack of motivation – you don't have a good enough reason to achieve your goals.
- A sense of purpose and being consistent – you swing wildly between bouts of feverish activity and none at all.
- Lack of persistence – you are too easily put off by lack of results.

## Willpower

Willpower needs direction. Hating yourself or the way you look is a powerful enough reason to take action, but the enormity of the task can sap your will. I can quite understand it, and the analogy which springs to my mind was when I had a new sophisticated computer system delivered just at a time when I was fiendishly busy on another project. To imagine that I could learn the ten thousand capabilities it had while my brain was already totally engaged elsewhere made me panic: I could never learn to use it; I would have to go on courses; stay up half the night; the office was small already and it was taking up half the room. Why hadn't I thought about all this when I bought it? I felt totally defeated by the enormity of the task ahead of me so I put the computer in another room, shut the door and pretended it didn't exist.

A week later and the scene had changed. A quiet afternoon meant a chance to clear the decks and assemble my computer. I'd bought it for databases and spreadsheets, so I decided to find out about those facilities for now, and leave the rest for later. I'd sorted out my priorities and suddenly the task wasn't so enormous. What this tells you about willpower in body chaos is that a task seems enormous if you don't sort out what you really want and if the stakes aren't that high. I didn't have to get the computer system sorted now, or ever. I'd bought it to help my systems, but the problem was that my systems were quite satisfactory as they stood. They just needed updating. I just didn't have the right incentive to embrace a course of computer training, so I abandoned it – at least until my mind was less stressed. This is why people find it hard to diet when they have a lot going on in their lives, like exams for example. I'm the first person to say that it doesn't take much time to eat less, but I accept that mental attitude needs psychological strength.

So sort out what you really want, in detail, and it won't seem such a massive task. Is it better legs, a flatter stomach, weight loss or what? Clear the decks one day, sit down and write out what you hate about yourself. Then write down what you hate about the way you live. It all comes back to successful living. Maybe you wouldn't have a figure problem if you didn't have to spend half your life driving. Perhaps all the corporate entertaining you get involved in means you're always tempted by food, and you hate this aspect of your job? A common unpopular lifestyle feature is 'having food in' – which tends to happen in families where snacks are thought to be necessary and available. Obviously a larder full of temptation is going to seriously dent your willpower during weak moments, but whatever your reasons for lack of willpower, lack of purpose and direction are usually high on the list.

## Motivation

Most people are motivated to do something about themselves when they have a special event looming, a holiday or scary photos which tell the full horror story of weight gain and lack of exercise! The difficulty is in maintaining that motivation. A little weight loss is usually enough to weaken resolve, and many people never reach their targets. The way to maintain motivation is to set goals, but never make weight loss a goal in itself, because you are then left with nothing to achieve once you have got there. A good motivation is another event, another holiday or even just a trip somewhere or a new dress. After all, it is all down to willpower!

## A Sense of Purpose

A sense of purpose is defined as 'the object for which something exists or is done'. You should therefore set your goals and ambitions in order of importance to you, and arrange your life to accommodate them. Being consistent is the next most important thing, and consistency is the ability to be free from irregularity – to be continuous and free of variation in the routine you set yourself. To do this, you must set yourself a life pattern that you know you can keep to realistically, for the rest of your life, and this means:

- A plan which is not beyond you physically
- A plan that involves doing the things you like doing
- A plan that you are temperamentally suited to e.g. not being with others when you are a loner by nature.

## Being Persistent

Being persistent is important. This means that you continue in spite of opposition, such as:

- From friends dissuading you – maybe because they envy your success
- Family making it difficult for you

Be fair with everyone, but expect fairness in return. It is not selfish to want to devote some time to yourself. It is not vain to want to get and hang on to a healthy, attractive figure. It is failing yourself and everybody else if you give way and lack persistence, and end up disappointed and depressed.

## Having a Plan

Many people are around food all the time, yet they don't eat until mealtimes, so I wonder what it is about some of us which makes us eat when we're not hungry, eat when we know we shouldn't and eat food we don't even particularly like?

If you are going out for a special evening meal, it's easy to refuse an afternoon tea. The dinner is inevitable and you must save your calories otherwise you'll get fat. What problem eaters do when faced with temptation is tell themselves that they can make up for it elsewhere. If you have that slice of apple pie and cream it won't really matter because you'll miss lunch. Then three o'clock comes and you haven't had anything since the apple pie and because you missed lunch you're hungry again. The cupboard has the usual tin of biscuits so you have a few with your coffee, then finish off those baked beans because you suddenly feel sickly. Maybe a slice of toast as well – oh, all right have two and don't have any supper. So everyone comes home and eats supper and you're having nothing. What you've ended up doing is having all snacks and no meals, but worse than that, your mind's been in chaos all day and you feel guilty.

People who eat properly do so because their meals are a fixture. They have a routine. They won't eat the apple pie because lunch is at 12.30. They won't have the afternoon biscuits because dinner's at 6.00 and even though they're hungry it's better to have an appetite because it's lamb chops tonight. So here I am telling you what slim people do and you might be thinking, 'So what? I'm not one of them' – but this is my point. There's not a special type of person who's slim. There are no qualifications required for having willpower. You need to think yourself into being that sort of person and you'll have the strength. Remember back in the introduction when I told you how I got over cigarettes by wondering what non-smokers thought when cigarettes came round? I promise you it isn't hard to imagine yourself a different person – we do it all the time when we dress up or go to an interview, so take the plunge! Give it a try for a week and see how nice it is to know you must have that lunch, you must have that dinner. You can't make up for your lapse by skipping it because it'll be on the table and you'll have to eat it. Have direction. Decide you're going to be healthy and slim, and you're going to stop the bad habit of only talking about your shortcomings all the time. You can!

Now all this might sound like such hard work that like my computer, you hide this book so you won't have to think about it. But it isn't a massive task. Take the example of wanting to lose 9.5kg, get rid of the fat on your hips and have shapelier calves. Here's how you might arrange it:

1. I'll go on a diet of 1400 calories a day, but I won't do it on a Sunday because we always enjoy lunch with mum.

2. I'm not going to aerobics or the gym because I can't stand

the distractions of others but I'll buy a video. I'm busy on Tuesdays and Thursday, but I can definitely slot in an hour on all the other days except Sunday.

3. My hips need extra toning. I'm not going for bike rides because the great outdoors just doesn't suit me, so I'll buy an exercise bike. I'll probably ride it for 30 minutes while *Coronation Street*'s on.

4. With 9.5kg to lose, I can manage about a kilo a week, so I'll set a date of 12 weeks to give me a bit of leeway.

5. My calves are dreadful – I'm going to measure them first so I know if they're getting any bigger, then do calf raises for three minutes after each workout, then measure them again after a month.

So what we have achieved here is:

- Not just saying you want something but defining EXACTLY what you want.
- Deciding how you intend doing it.
- Giving a timeframe.
- Setting points to assess your progress.

## Mental Gremlins

Many forgotten snacks happen as part of an activity, even eating a slice of toast while you're on the phone. You might think that you won't enjoy these activities if you don't eat at the same time as doing them, but you will. There is nothing about food which actually makes these activities more pleasant – they are good in themselves. You need to unlearn the association and the activities will be just as pleasant as before.

You might have found that food has become your best friend and even a part of your personality. You might be a great cook, wonderful mother or simply great fun when out for a meal. Like a friend, food is always there for you, it perks you up when you're down, it's part of your daily life. However you need to remember that it's not really your best friend – your best friend wouldn't make you look and feel so bad!

We've all got weak spots, but be honest about why you eat. Some people feel guilty, others get depressed or angry, but most women simply come to the conclusion that they are weak and somehow different from everyone else. Here are some examples of mental gremlins:

1. *'How can one biscuit hurt?'*

   This first gremlin tells you to go ahead and have a biscuit because you will stop at just one.

2. *'Everything kills you these days. Why should I diet when I could be run over by a bus tomorrow?'*

   This gremlin tells you that compared with an accident, your eating habits are trivial. It plays down the consequences, while ignoring the fact that you really wish you could stick to a diet. The outcome of giving in to gremlins is never happy.

## Confronting Those Gremlins

### The 'I feel wonderful' gremlin

Telling yourself how wonderful life is with food is completely opposite to reality.

'One cake won't hurt.'

'I'm enjoying myself – I'm not going to spoil it by denying myself.'

### The truth

You are caught in believing that this wonderful time will somehow be better if you eat twice as much. You know that if you control yourself, you'll feel great tomorrow and if you don't, you'll end up depressed and angry with yourself, and it will only put off the day when you have to address your weight again.

### The 'I feel terrible' gremlin

This is the one where you tell yourself that you are weak and bound to fail, and that dieting isn't worth it anyway.

'I'm just a bundle of nerves.'

'Diets never work for me.'

'I'm just a weak person like my mother.'

### The truth

This gremlin is a making-mountains-out-of-molehills one, like chucking up a good job for a trivial reason, ending a relationship just because he snores. It is most active when you are in danger of a relapse, so focus on the reality. Feeling the way you do right now might not seem worth being hungry, but it goes off. Get past this moment with a milky drink, and concentrate on the real reason you're dieting.

### The best friend gremlin

This one makes you feel that your relationship with food is a friend.

'When I stop for a coffee it just isn't the same without a biscuit.'

'A drive in the country isn't the same without a pub meal.'

'Meeting friends is better if we can have lunch.'

### The truth

Food is always there as a comfort, like a best friend. But remember that you can still enjoy these activities without food, and does comfort-eating really comfort you? How do you really feel afterwards?

## The 'oppressed minority' gremlin

This gremlin is the one which gives you the status of an oppressed minority with your rights being taken away.

'I choose to be fat – women should be allowed to be the shape they want to be!'

### The truth

This is fine if you really feel this way, but genuinely happy women rarely feel the need to fight their corner – they just shrug it off. By taking on the mantle of an oppressed minority such people somehow feel they can hide behind their 'rights' which then can take the responsibility away from them.

## Getting The Better of the Gremlins

### Get beyond this moment

If you are simply craving a piece of chocolate, hunk of cheese or whatever, and you know that it will trigger a major relapse, concentrate very hard on getting through this moment to the other side. You should do something else, drink a glass of water, get out of the house for a moment. Don't eat – even if it's only a 'healthy' food like a few grapes. Never satisfy a food craving if you aren't really hungry and in need of your next meal. Concentrate on the time for your next meal and think of how you imagine yourself looking in a coveted outfit. You'll get through.

### Don't let self-hate get the better of you

The self-hate gremlin happens to everyone, but it's not true that you're just a weak, hopeless person. Remember, gremlins are really just another side of you, the frightened bit of your mind who fears that you really might be hopeless – so you try and get in first. You can certainly be weak at times just like anyone else, but that doesn't mean to say you are weak. Just remember that if you're having a blue day, scoffing a fattening meal isn't going to make it any better.

### Get some new friends

This is hard, but for the time being you must stop seeing people who are gremlins themselves! Stop going to all the places where your gremlins hang out because otherwise the habit will become impossible to break. Find some new coffee shops or restaurants because even the sight of the familiar wallpaper will encourage you to choose that bun or those biscuits. Ask someone else to pick up your children from school, go to work using a different route. It might be inconvenient to start with, but man is a hunter, hunters are territorial and territory comes with a set of markers. Friends are a way of marking out the boundaries of your life and they might be bad for you just now. Start a new routine, tell people why you're doing this, and if you're associating with people who have bad habits themselves, give them the elbow. Being around fit, healthy people will be your best incentive to stay on track.

### Face up to your lapses

Eating is not like being an alcoholic where one drink is one drink too many. Try to take a relapse as an isolated one, and not begin to catastrophize the consequences into being a total failure as a human being!

## The Good News About Adopting New Eating Habits

- Eating less pays. If you have been buying fast food, extra cakes or crisps and having second helpings, the saving will be immense. In a single year you will save enough for a holiday!

- You will gain years of life by reducing heart disease and lowering blood pressure.
- You will reduce the pressure on your knees and hips.
- You will feel better about yourself.
- You will be able to wear the clothes you really like.

In short, you have everything to gain and nothing to lose if you start a healthy, weight-loss diet!

## Realistic Expectations

To overcome your body chaos properly, I can't emphasize enough how important it is to draw a line under your old life and start again. Don't look back on past failures, but look ahead. This is your body, and you want it to be well, healthy and attractive.

The image of the overweight woman is that she is fat from childhood, ignorant of good eating habits, idle and indulgent. Some are, but many are not. Most people I deal with are smart, professional women who have enjoyed the best in life, worn designer clothes and pride themselves on never having a hair out of place or a rogue inch on their waistlines. They might be in their early twenties used to the compliments that come with being a head-turning teenager or a new mother. They might be approaching the menopause. Whatever their place in life, they are used to being in control of their looks, but this time they're beaten. Why are their hormones playing up, and why can't they stop the weight piling on?

Well, I can't always help with hormones especially if

there's a problem with them and you need medical advice, but I need to start with a realistic look at how much weight you should expect to lose when you go on a diet. Expectation is important: if you think you should be losing 3kg a week and you only lose just over a kilo, you feel a failure. If you expect to lose under a kilo and you lose just over a kilo, you've exceeded your expectations.

So, to start with the facts, I asked Professor John Garrow to help. He ran obesity clinics for the NHS for twenty-four years, and studied the patients admitted to his metabolic ward. They were clinically obese, and had tried and repeatedly failed to lose weight on standard regimes. They were admitted to the ward so that their eating habits and metabolic rates could be studied in more detail.

Half a kilo of fat is equal to 3,850 calories (a pound of fat is equal to 3,500 calories). It is reasonable to assume that on a calorie-deficient diet of 1,000 calories a day, you would lose 907g in weight, but it isn't like this. Gender and age come into the equation, but even more important is the condition of the person when he or she comes in. Here are some facts:

- Women tend to lose 1.03kg /week. Men lose 1.07kg/week.
- If the energy deficit is 1,000 calories a day there will be a 1kg/week weight loss after the first week but in the first week it is unpredictable, the average weight loss being 3.8kg in 3 weeks.
- If oedematous on admission (retaining water), weight loss can be rapid, with up to 5.5kg lost in the first week.
- If dehydrated (ketotic) on admission – in the first week and on a 1,000 calories a day deficit, the patient will *gain* weight. When rehydrated, the ketotic patients took an average of thirteen days to return to admission weight. Thereafter weight loss continued as predicted.
- Body weight versus body fat in women – for every 0.454kg of fat gained there is a weight increase of 0.57kg.

So you have to have realistic expectations of your weight loss, and be aware of what weight is. It is weight, not necessarily fat. On the bright side, adding exercise to your plan can make inroads into those muscles, and change your shape considerably. Indeed, exercise is the only way to change your shape significantly.

And are you giving yourself a fair chance? Three weeks is not enough time to see changes. Remember, all your body processes of growth and repair take about the same length of time. Skin takes a month to renew itself, hair takes three days to grow just one millimetre, so muscles aren't suddenly going to spring into shape.

## Your Plan of Action

1. Have a complete week off both diet and exercise. Eat what you want, relax. This way you'll be more than ready to make a fresh start.

2. Completely change your workout routine if you've been doing the same thing for more than two months. If you have been heavily into cardiovascular exercise and feel worn out, give it a rest and spend more time with weights.

3. You must change the order of your meals, and the type of meal you are having. For example, if you always have a small lunch and bigger evening meal, swap them around. It might just be the breakthrough you need.

4. If you haven't already done so, measure everything. You need to see where, if anywhere, your fat is being lost from. Fat is usually lost from (in this order): the face, and chest, the abdominal cavity, between your shoulder blades and lastly off your hips.

5. Get up an hour earlier and do your aerobic routine. If you are doing weight training, the best time is between 4 and 6 p.m.

## Keeping Pace With Your Changing Metabolism

A muscle's job is to move your bones so you can make a movement of some sort. Muscles have enzymes working in them all the time to keep up the turnover of normal degeneration and growth. Even if you are sitting doing nothing, your muscles are being serviced and kept in peak condition, rather like a car being cleaned and polished ready for its next outing. Muscle increases your resting metabolic rate because it is constantly degenerating and being rebuilt. The bad news about muscle is that it steadily decreases from about your mid-twenties onwards through normal ageing changes (and you thought twenty-five was young!). Although this erosion is only about 2 per cent every decade, the years can wear away without you realizing it. This 2 per cent means you need about 200 calories a day fewer by the time you are in your late fifties than you did in your mid-twenties, and although this doesn't sound very much, it's 73,000 calories a year – a staggering 9.5kg gained without you feeling that you've done anything to deserve it!

The current recommendation for a woman's daily calorie intake is 2,000, but I feel that this is way too high these days, when modern life has made us all a lot better off. We're not as cold as people used to be, for example, and we don't have to boil our clothes and scrub floors. I suggest no more than 1,800 calories a day by the time you reach sixty.

## Some of Your Excuses for Giving Up

Most of the people who contact me for diet advice, do so because they have exhausted every avenue open to them. They follow all the advice, do what they have always done, and get nowhere. I believe that there is always a way round everything, and if you go back right to the beginning of this book, you'll remember that life doesn't stand still. You do almost nothing now that you did as a girl – so why do you think your body is going to behave the same way? Here are some of your most frequent complaints:

### Eating Low-Fat Foods Makes No Difference

'I've always eaten low-fat, but now I'm still stuck at this weight. I thought I was doing the right thing.'

There is this complete myth about eating fat which is nonsense. If everyone who ate butter and cream and nuts was fat I could understand it, but they're not. It isn't a matter of luck, either. I could devise a complete eating plan without so much as a milligram of fat in it, and you could still gain weight. Meringues, boiled sweets, jam, fatless sponge, sweet pickle, brown sauce, instant mashed potatoes – put together they supply less than a tenth of a gram of fat, but they pack a huge calorie punch which can send your daily allowances sky high.

It's important to keep your total intake of fat at about 70g a day, with saturated fat (mostly animal fat) down to no more than 21g a day (look at food labels) and that's for health reasons. The trick is to eat meals which are low in fat overall, but not devoid of small amounts of the fats you like. It is better to limit yourself to a pat of butter every day on your toast if you really like it (10g portion = 5.4g of saturated fat) and eat fresh fish, vegetables, rice, pasta and fruit for your main meals, than to eat as much low-fat spread as you like in the belief that it is OK to do so. See how these add up:

- 4x14g portions of low-fat spread:     3.4g saturated fat
- low-fat crisps:                        2.8g saturated fat
- reduced-fat prawn sandwich:            3.0g saturated fat
- portion of low-fat Cheddar cheese:     8.7g saturated fat

All commendably under your day's maximum saturated fat allowance at about 18g, but an interesting 572 calories-worth of actual food. My point is this: would you have eaten the crisps or the sandwich or four servings of the full-fat products if there were no lower-fat versions on the market? You would probably go without, thus saving yourself a lot of calories.

I am not at all suggesting that you are being in some way naive or fooled by low-fat products, but I think they promise more than they can come up with. If you are trying to keep fat low for health reasons then this is the way to do it, but if you are trying to lose weight for a better figure, remember to count calories.

However, fat is important at every meal because along with protein, it slows down the rate at which your carbohydrates are absorbed. A salad sandwich is just carbohydrates, water, vitamins and minerals, with only a small amount of protein in the bread. A jacket potato and salad is also a virtually fat- and protein-free meal, which is why you might feel hungry a lot sooner after you've eaten them. Always add something like tuna fish, chicken, ham or cheese to your sandwiches, and you'll find your hunger is satisfied for longer.

## Cutting Out Sugar and Alcohol Make No Difference

'I've cut out sugar and alcohol and my weight's the same.'

This is really the same as the low-fat foods. In theory, if

you were consuming 300 calories a day in alcohol and sweets and you stopped having them, you could expect to lose just over a kilo. I've known a lot of stunning weight-loss successes from people who stuck to this regime for months, but it doesn't usually work like that. Instead of a tube of Smarties (170 calories) you munch on a couple of apples (100 calories): you say no to a glass of wine (95 calories) and yes to some fresh orange juice (57 calories).

The point is that if you're going to cut out something, leave the space, don't fill it with something else.

You shouldn't worry unduly about sugar as long as you control it. Don't munch on sweets because they damage your teeth, and don't buy sweetened breakfast cereals because you can't control the amount of sugar that is in them. But if you like a teaspoon of sugar on your cereal, have it – I do! If ever you go to a gathering you'll notice that the people taking a couple of sugars in their coffee are generally the slimmest in the room, and the ones daintily waving away the puddings and nibbling round the outside of an after-dinner mint are usually the fattest – and doing a lot of their eating in private. If you accept chocolate and puddings as part of normal life, you won't crave them and you won't have a weight problem. Sweet things aren't 'treats' – they're normal food. A calorie is a calorie after all, and a few calories from sugar once a day won't do you any harm. If you're intent on losing weight take a broad-brush approach and first remove calories which you don't notice or appreciate – you did that by ditching alcohol and sweets – and then cut down on portion sizes. Above all, exercise as much as you can, and get a proper breakfast every day.

### I Don't Eat Breakfast, But I Don't Lose Weight

'I never eat breakfast – I just can't face food first thing and if I start eating then, I'll eat for the rest of the day.'

I could buy this argument if it seemed to work, but most people who claim that not eating breakfast keeps their appetites in check are not usually good advertisements for this philosophy. It just doesn't wash. In one study it was found that people who missed breakfast ate more at lunch, and those who fasted all day ate the biggest evening meal, thus cancelling out any calorie benefits. People who believe that eating somehow 'sets them off' are playing a game with food which is more about psychology and control. Eating breakfast reduces the desire to eat a lot later on, whereas the hunger level is driven up the longer you leave it. Many people also report that they go a whole day 'forgetting' to eat, but this is not true. I have found that such people keep hunger pangs at bay with sweet drinks, sweets, the odd biscuit and so on. You can't go without food for eight hours and not feel hungry. So eat breakfast, eat lunch and eat again in the evening.

### What's the Point When I Stay at the Same Weight?

'I've dieted for years and after a few weeks I just stick at the same weight. Why does this "plateau" happen?'

According to Professor John Garrow, the mid-diet plateau does exist, but it is not explained by a decrease in metabolic rate. Hundreds of patients were referred to Professor Garrow by their GPs because they were experiencing this plateau. When they were admitted to the metabolic ward and ate exactly the same diet on which they had been previously losing weight, they lost weight again. When their metabolic rate was measured, it was what could be expected for their weight and body composition.

When a person first starts to diet they lose weight rather quickly, because they lose muscle glycogen and water. After a week or so this runs out, and weight loss is then mainly 75 per cent fat and 25 per cent non-fat tissue (muscle) – and this takes a lot longer to be used as it is more dense. Therefore on the diet the rate of weight loss decreases.

Your metabolic rate does decrease as weight is lost at the rate of about 12 cals/day for each kilo lost in women and 16 cals/kg/day for men. Therefore, for a woman to lose 10kg she would either need to eat 120 calories a day fewer or increase exercise every day to get rid of 120 calories – either way not a demanding regime. However, overweight people start off with a higher metabolic rate than lean people of the same age, gender and height, so after initial weight loss their metabolic rate would have decreased to a normal level not below normal! How come overweight people have a higher metabolism? Simple. Like a big car with a big engine which needs more petrol than a small car, if you have to drag about a body which weighs, for arguments' sake, 114 kilos, this is a considerable effort for your body. The lean woman of about 44 kilos has less than half the weight to move around, so consequently her metabolic rate will be lower. The difference would be between about 50 calories an hour for the thin person but 102 calories an hour, more than double for the overweight person.

So how come people experience a complete stop in their weight loss – the so-called plateau? Professor Garrow explains it thus, 'Patients think I am accusing them of lying about what they eat, or being too stupid to calculate their diet. This is not true: I am saying that many people do not recall accurately what they eat, just as I do not recall accurately what I have spent on cash purchases. This does not make me either dishonest or stupid, but it does mean that when I am asked what I have spent in the last few days I cannot give an accurate reply, because I do not know the correct amount.'

So the answer to beating the weight-loss plateau is to stick rigidly to your diet, observing weights, measures and portion sizes religiously, and taking into account the slight decrease in the calories your body needs as you get lighter. This needn't lead to an obsessive state of weighing and calculating everything every time you eat, but an awareness of your meals, and an awareness of whether or not you are beginning to slacken off, exercise less, or generally getting complacent about your goals.

## I Don't Eat Much But I'm Not Losing Weight

'I eat very little all day and like to look forward to a nice main meal in the evening – but I still can't shift this weight.'

I can see the logic behind this – you want something to look forward to at the end of the day, especially something which can be shared as a family meal. However, eating large numbers of calories at a time when you're going to be relaxing is a bad idea. You can still sit and enjoy a meal with everyone else, but why don't you all have a light meal like salad or fish and vegetables followed by something sweet but light, such as mousse or stewed fruit? If you are on a weight-loss diet you should have three meals a day with the same number of calories (400) and two energy breaks of 150 calories.

## I Don't Eat in the Evening But I Still Don't Lose Weight

'I try not to eat after 6 p.m. because calories eaten in the evening just turn straight to fat.'

This is completely untrue, and I see no point in trying not to eat in the evening unless it suits you. If you really have a problem with boredom setting in, you should save your last meal as something to look forward to at about 9–9.30 p.m. There is no truth in the old wives' tale about eating late causing fat to settle more easily, especially as your body doesn't know what time it is. Make sure your last meal is a low glycaemic index one and does not contain any red meat, (as this takes eight hours to digest), or fat and starch together as in pastry or cakes.

## It's Too Difficult to Have a Routine

'I can't eat regularly because I never know where I'll be from one day to the next.'

Plan your journey and itinerary around the mealbreak, not the other way round. Tell yourself that you'll need to stop at 12.30 p.m., and programme the alarm in your wristwatch or whatever, to remind you. If you're hungry before that time, wait. Whatever you do, don't respond instantly to those first few hunger pangs with the first thing that comes to hand, steering the car erratically, dropping crumbs and goodness' knows what else into your lap as you wrestle with a titanic baguette. Be rigid in your set times of feeding and get your body used to routine. Can't be bothered? Think I don't understand about deadlines, traffic chaos and the problems of having to work through your breaks? Well, you don't have to take my advice, but aren't you desperate to change?

## I Turned Fifty and Gained Twelve Kilos Immediately!

Although this sounds like a tabloid headline, it's actually similar to the first sentence of lots of letters I receive on a weekly basis. It seems impossible that so many people can have the same experience, but weight gain and middle age seem to go together like Rogers and Hammerstein or tea and biscuits. But is it really a foregone conclusion or one of those old chestnuts? Times have changed, and with the average age for motherhood now standing at thirty-one and many teenagers topping the scales heavier than their grannies, old ideas need a re-think. Isn't it time to ditch our old prejudices about what happens to our bodies in middle age?

Centuries ago, women didn't experience the menopause as we do because most of them were dead by the time it would have struck. Lack of recreational exercise, severe physical deformities as a result of childbirth and unbalanced nutrition for even the wealthiest women, meant that for those who survived, old age began early. And after all, what would most of us look like if we had no hair dyes, tweezers for taming eyebrows, face creams or make-up? It doesn't bear thinking about. Even our grandmothers and mothers would have considered forty to be the age when a little gentle keep fit might be attempted, as long as it wasn't strenuous. The only super-fit middle-aged women would have been former athletes or dancers and, as such, an exception to the rule. This is not to say that 'ordinary' women did not keep fit. Women were as likely to hike and ride for pleasure as they were to labour long and hard in factories, but for those who worked, exercise was repetitive and a strain on the body, often leaving a legacy of back pain, muscular strain and bone weakness. Exercise for looks and beauty was not unknown, but it did not become part of the popular culture until comparatively recently. In the twenty-first century it's a different scene. Women approaching forty or fifty can have an impressive twenty years of aerobics, weight-training, boxercise, Pilates, yoga and gym culture under their belts, and they come from all walks of life. Compared with the younger generation they are the true masters and authorities on physical fitness, so anyone treating fifty-year-olds as shuffling old women exercising at half the pace of teenagers is displaying a woeful ignorance. After all, if you are a twenty-five-year-old fitness fanatic how would you feel if at the age of fifty you were treated by some youngster as a total beginner needing to go half the speed of younger class members?

So, back to gaining two stone at the age of fifty. Yes, anybody can gain weight alarmingly quickly if they don't keep tabs on themselves. No, there isn't anything magical about this age. After all, your brain doesn't understand birthdays. Your body hasn't a clue you're fifty years old, and all your body chemistry does is react to a set of hormones and other circumstances which dictate your metabolism, weight and physical condition.

## Your Plan of Action

1. Keep tabs on your weight. Anyone can gain a few kilos without noticing or being worried, but you should monitor these big weight gains and take steps before the task that faces you gets too enormous. Sometimes people will say to me, 'I seem to have gained nineteen kilos (three stone) and I can't understand it.' I can understand missing a few rogue kilos, I can even see how you can be a bit preoccupied and ignore an extra 5kg or so but 19kg!! Try as I might, I can't see why someone would not take steps before this stage was reached.

2. When you are young I advise weighing yourself no more than once a month – when you reach the change you should weigh yourself weekly and take steps if the increase is more than 1.5kg, (a normal daily weight fluctuation).

3. Realize how your life has shifted in the past 20–30 years. You might think that you live as you have always done, but the changes in your routine are subtle. If you always used to walk the children just five minutes to the bus, carry your shopping home or wash dishes by hand, and now your children have left home, you drive to the shops and you have a dishwasher, this can mean between 300–500 calories a day you aren't using up any longer. These changes rarely happen at the same time, but unless you replace them with another activity, the weight can creep on. 300 calories a day is 9,000 a month. About half a kilo of excess fat accumulates when you are 3,500 calories in excess, so this would mean a weight gain of about 1.5kg a month, about 13kg in a year, everything being equal.

People will tell me that they eat the same and are as active as they ever were, and that this weight gain is totally mystifying. You can't gain about 13kg 'immediately', but you can certainly gain it without realizing, especially when you believe that nothing in your life has altered to any great degree. The examples I have just given are a good indicator of how small changes in routine have a significant effect on your weight.

4. Build up muscle. This sounds depressingly like starting a bodybuilding course, but it isn't. Having a good amount of muscle on your body will do more for your weight than any diet will ever achieve. This is because muscle is metabolically active, it does a job and needs servicing even if you are lying in bed asleep. As we all get older our muscles automatically decrease in size and although this sounds contradictory, the weight loss from lack of muscle mass is more than made up by the weight GAIN from the slower metabolism. So keep doing the aerobics but don't concentrate on burning calories to the exclusion of weight training.

5. Eat 200 calories a day fewer. A good rule of thumb is that you need about 200 calories a day fewer by the time you reach fifty – (increase that to 220 by the age of seventy which might seem too slight a distinction, but which is 7,300 a year – another kilo gained!) An alternative piece of advice would be to burn an extra 200 calories in exercise, and this is good too, but I find that it is more reliable to plan a daily menu where items are simply reduced. An example might be to reduce two biscuits to one, change milk from semi-skimmed to skimmed and stop taking sugar in hot drinks. Reducing portion size is another easy way to do this.

## Hormone Replacement Therapy

Many women experience weight gain on HRT, but there is nothing in it which actually alters your balance of energy. As you know, fat is stored as a result of a calorie imbalance. Younger women also report weight gain on the contraceptive Pill, but there seems to be no correlation between these hormones and weight gain, otherwise everyone who took them would automatically gain weight.

Indeed, according to Dr Beverley Carey of the Centre for Nutritional Medicine, with the right HRT therapy many women actually lose weight as their metabolisms return to that of their younger years. Oestrogen definitely causes a redistribution of fat away from the abdominal region and onto the breasts and buttocks, thereby presenting a slimmer, more youthful waistline. So don't get involved in too many scare stories about HRT. It might be just what you need.

## Weight Gain in General Mid-life

There is absolutely no reason why you can't keep your youthful figure well into old age. I truly believe that if you decide that middle-age spread is inevitable, it will be. If you are determined to keep your figure, you will. It might not be possible to exercise in exactly the same way as you used to, but by substituting other forms of exercise you can stay flexible, supple, strong and toned. There is no difference to the chemistry of fat storage and energy balance as you get older, but it is stored slightly differently. The dwindling oestrogen in midlife means that testosterone comes to the fore. Testosterone isn't a hormone I have talked about before because women have only small amounts of it and it is effectively a male hormone, but when testosterone is not masked by oestrogen it comes dominant, and you gain weight in the male pattern. You also get more facial hair, a slightly deeper voice and become more assertive, which can't be a bad thing. So the menopause puts weight distribution down to an android figure rather than the hourglass figure of the gynoid – fat on legs and hips. You might say, 'ten years ago I weighed "this" and now I weigh the same but I've got this huge stomach.' But remember that the stomach doesn't come out of the blue. Anticipate the changes! So . . . keep up with the little jobs – control the changes, have some discipline in your exercise habits, and remember to respect yourself! You deserve it.

## How You Can Beat the Clock

1. Don't leave it all too late. If you were the teenager who thought that smoking damage wouldn't happen to you, now's the time you'll see those puckered lips and poor skin quality. Nicotine is a poison. If you are smoking at the moment, it's not too late to stop and see the benefits.

2. Heed the warnings about sunbathing. People will claim that they moisturize well before and after tanning, or use a high-protection factor sunscreen, but if you have achieved a change in the colour of your skin and are even a little tanned, damage has occurred. Use a fake tan.

3. Exercise aerobically, weight train and introduce a good stretch routine. A youthful body is a supple one.

4. Wear a good bra: youth means a high bustline. Youth means silky hair which gleams and moves when you walk and talk. Youth is about doing things quickly or with gusto – even talking quickly, looking animated, laughing a lot. People who walk in a laboured way, talk without energy, slouch, complain a lot and don't smile much, can be mistaken for older than their true age.

# Chapter Eight

# Before Your Weight-Loss Plan

## Your Basic Daily Calorie Requirements

Weight loss should be achieved through fat burning in exercise, with a corresponding calorie deficit of 500 a day.

This is how to calculate a very rough estimate of your metabolic rate (BMR), but it is impossible to know your exact metabolic rate unless you spend a night in a metabolic ward. But this estimate is quite good enough because it takes your age into account.

Wkg means your weight in kilograms, and if you are still working to pounds and stones, simply multiply your weight in pounds by 2.2 to find the kilograms.

| Age Range | Kcal (min) |
| --- | --- |
| 10–17 years | $13.4 \times Wkg + 692 = ?$ |
| 18–28 years | $14.8 \times Wkg + 487 = ?$ |
| 30–59 years | $8.3 \times Wkg + 846 = ?$ |

Example: a woman, aged 23, who weighs 58 kilos.
BMR = $14.8 \times 58 = 858.4$
$858 + 487 = 1345$ calories per day

Example: a girl, aged 15, who weighs 58 kilos.
BMR = $13.4 \times 58 = 772$
$772 + 692 = 1464$ calories.

## Maximum Calories Needed Per Day

| Age Range | Calories |
| --- | --- |
| 11–14 years | 1845 |
| 15–18 years | 2110 |
| 19–50 years | 1940 |
| 51–59 years | 1990 |
| 60–64 years | 1990 |
| 65–74 years | 1990 |
| 75+ years | 1810 |

So from these calculations you can see that if you are an average fifteen-year-old you would need a minimum of 1464 calories a day at this weight, and a maximum of 2110 calories. If you are a fifty-three-year-old woman also weighing 66 kilos your ideal calorie recommendation would be from 1393 calories to 1990 calories.

You will also see from the tables that while calorie needs for teenagers are undoubtedly higher than for seniors, they are not that much higher! The difference in recommended daily intakes between a sixty-five-year-old and an eighteen-year-old is just 200 calories a day, so if anyone is feeding you up with lashings of butter on your sandwiches and a double helping of pudding 'because you're growing', they're not doing you any favours!

## Energy Balance

Energy balance is as simple as a bank balance. If the calories in your food are used up by your body, you won't have any left over to be stored as fat. If you have more calories than you are using on a regular basis the excess will be stored as fat.

To appreciate simple energy balance, take a look at this perfectly ordinary food and activity account of a normal woman who could be you.

This activity diary has been kept for us by a forty-one-year-old woman called Christine. She weighs 67.7 kilos, and is 157cm tall. She works in an office, travels to work by car which is parked directly outside and she spends 3–4 hours at a time sitting at a computer. When home, she prepares meals for herself and her husband. She says she is too tired after her daily journey home for formal exercise; she is also dissatisfied with the shape of her legs, midriff and back. In particular, Christine is worried about 'creeping' weight gain and joint stiffness. She is blaming her hormones.

| Activity | Cal/min | Total Calories |
| --- | --- | --- |
| Sleeping, 7 hours | 1 | 420 |
| Washing and dressing, 30 minutes | 2 | 60 |
| Eating breakfast, 20 minutes | 1.5 | 30 |
| Driving to work, 45 minutes | 1.5 | 68 |
| Office work, sitting, 9–12.30 p.m. | 1.5 | 315 |
| Walk to shops and back, 30 minutes | 4 | 120 |
| Office work, sitting 1.00–5.30 p.m. | 1.5 | 405 |
| Drive home, 55 minutes | 0.5 | 83 |
| Cooking and eating, 60 minutes | 1.5 | 90 |
| Ironing and tidying, 30 minutes | 2.5 | 75 |
| Watching TV, 4 hours | 1.5 | 360 |
| TOTAL | | 2026 |

Christine also kept a food diary for us. She keeps to healthy, no-additive food, deliberately choosing low-fat, sugar-free alternatives to standard foods. On this day she allowed herself her usual 'treat' of half a Twirl bar after lunch.

| Time | Food | Calories | |
|------|------|---------:|--|
| 7.30 a.m. | 40g Bran Flakes, no sugar | 130 | |
| | 150ml semi-skimmed milk | 62 | |
| | 2 cups coffee semi-skimmed milk | 40 | |
| | 150ml orange 'just juice' | 65 | |
| | | | **297 calories** |
| 10.30 a.m. | Nutri-grain bar | 140 | |
| | carton pure apple juice | 65 | |
| | | | **350 calories** |
| 12.30 p.m. | free-range egg & cress roll | 410 | |
| | fresh fruit salad, 397g pack | 195 | |
| | one finger Twirl | 115 | |
| | 2 cups coffee, milk | 40 | |
| | | | **760 calories** |
| 3.15 p.m. | apple | 55 | |
| | cup tea | 20 | |
| | glass water | nil | |
| | | | **85 calories** |
| 6.40 p.m. | nibble of bread, peanut butter | 120 | |
| | cup tea | 20 | |
| | | | *140 calories* |
| 7.30 p.m. | jacket potato, 226g | 200 | |
| | stir-fried chicken breast, dsp oil | 220 | |
| | broccoli and peas | 55 | |
| | 4 sips someone else's wine (half glass) | 50 | |
| | glass water | nil | |
| | raspberry healthy eating yoghurt | 60 | |
| | 2 cups coffee | 40 | |
| | | | **625 calories** |
| 9.30 p.m. | low-fat hot chocolate drink | 40 | |
| | apple | 55 | |
| | 1 reduced-fat digestive biscuit | 70 | |
| | | | **165 calories** |
| | **GRAND TOTAL** | | **2277 calories** |

Deficit on the day 2277–2026 = 251 calories
Over 7 days = 1757 calories
Over a month = 7028 calories = 900g
Over a year = 91,615 calories = 11.8kg!

Now of course it doesn't work like this, because food intake and exercise vary. At weekends you are more likely to go for a walk, go dancing, do the garden or simply catch up on bits round the house – in any event you are unlikely to be sitting on your backside for seven hours on a Saturday – or are you? But the downside is that you might also eat a lot more. A Sunday roast, tea with your auntie, a bottle of wine on Saturday night – this is how you send your calories rocketing. So my suggestions to help Christine deal with her weight gain and joint stiffness are simple: extra exercise in the evening instead of watching four hours of television! This would deal with all her problems at once without her having to cut out any of her favourite food, and I also recommended her buying an exercise bike to put in the spare bedroom so she wouldn't even have to leave home. The result? Christine lost a steady kilo in weight a week for eight weeks and her hormones seem to have settled down. By adding a stretch session at the end of her exercise routine, she feels less stiff and is sleeping better.

## I Don't Know Where to Start

We weren't all brought up knowing how to manage a home and cooking. I come from an academic family, with a mother who would rather we practised playing the piano than learn to cook, and indeed she was not a good cook herself. Like many people, therefore, I was launched into the adult world without a clue where to start, so here are the major areas of difficulty for people new to managing their diet for themselves:

- portion sizes
- eating on the run
- cooking methods like frying
- snacking automatically in front of the TV etc.
- eating wherever it is convenient
- food being used as a reward

It's not just what you should eat, but what you look for in the shops and how you cook it. Part of the mental chaos over food is in thinking of random bits of food which you either like or hate and not quite knowing what to do with them. I've given you a reasonable teenagers' diet on page 223, but here are the sort of things you should look out for:

- fresh chicken breasts – buy 2–4 at a time
- boil-in-the bag cod and parsley sauce
- tinned mixed beans
- tinned tomatoes with onions and peppers etc.
- dried pasta shapes
- plain Basmati rice
- brown pudding rice (short grain)
- tinned sweetcorn
- frozen peas
- fresh apples, bananas, grapes etc.
- muesli
- dried fruit
- packet sunflower seeds
- mixed nuts

## Planning Your Meals

The best way to plan meals is to get as much preparation done in one go as possible. Another good idea is to cook by what I call my 'one spare' system. This means that when you cook, say, a chicken breast for your evening meal, you cook another one at the same time and leave it in the fridge, cold, ready for a sandwich or salad the next day. Here are some other ideas for saving time:

- Fill the oven with several items which can cook together such as two fillets of fish, chicken portions, etc.
- Make a very large rice pudding using 2.25 litres (4pt) milk – pot up into small dishes, cover with clingfilm and you have enough for a week.
- Make a large container of mixed salad on Sunday evening which will see you through the week.
- Have stir-fry mixed vegetables ready-prepared.
- Hard-boil 2 or 3 eggs, ready for salads or sandwiches.
- Boil and cool a few potatoes, mix with a little mayonnaise and leave covered in the fridge as potato salad.
- Mix up your own high-energy muesli adding nuts, seeds and extra dried fruit to shop-bought unsweetened muesli. Take to work or school in an airtight container, adding milk and plain yoghurt.

Being successful on a healthy eating plan means being prepared. Most bad eating habits start because you're short of time, for example, you're just home on a freezing winter's night, there's only a piece of frozen meat in your fridge and nothing to go with it. Then it's either off to the takeaway or out with the cheese and biscuits, and we all know where that leads. Eating quickly to satisfy real hunger can mean that you take on board far more calories than you really want, simply because you don't feel full for twenty minutes. The alternative scenario of course is that you take time to thaw the meat and peel some potatoes – but while they're cooking you satisfy your hunger with a packet of crisps, a bite of that cake going stale in the tin and two squares of chocolate. But it's a winning situation if you can simply have the makings of your meal ready to pop into a pan.

In the recipe section I've given you several incredibly quick ideas for stir-fries or grills which can be on the table in less than ten minutes. The best news is that they're all nutritious, low in calories and best of all, unprocessed. Remember that processed, refined food comes with the warning that it can seriously affect your moods and energy levels, so make a promise to yourself that you'll start to cook for yourself properly in future, and overcome your body chaos into the bargain.

## Eating Habits

'I have terrible eating habits – and my stomach feels bloated and painful into the bargain.'

Well then, what you should do is:

- Always have breakfast, and make sure you have enough calories in the morning, even if you are going to be sitting down all day.
- Eat three hours later, a small low glycaemic index snack such as oatcakes, bananas or cereal, for a fuller list see the glycaemic index on page 304.
- Lunch should be substantial in content but not size as you have a long 'haul' to the end of the day and your next main meal. Have some high or intermediate glycaemic index foods like potatoes or pasta, with protein and some vegetables or salad.
- Your mid-afternoon slump can be cured with two pieces of fruit, and this will also give you vital water which stops you feeling tired.
- Your evening meal should always be light, unless you are planning to go out

and do other activities. If it is winter and you plan to relax, have a light salad with protein, and fresh fruit.

- Your last meal should be light and calming, so warm milk and banana, a small portion of rice pudding, yoghurt with dried fruit or cereal is ideal.

## Poor Eating Habits, Such As?

- Eating standing up, eating in the car, eating in the street, eating while preparing food.
- Eating with fingers, not cutlery.
- 'Fork loading' – loading the next mouthful while you are still chewing the first one.
- Not chewing properly. Swallowing big lumps of food causes wind and indigestion – often assumed to be a food intolerance!
- Diving into pudding the minute your main course is finished.

## What Should I Do?

- Never go shopping when you are hungry – you will have low blood sugar by the time you've finished shopping and will tear into the first bag you can to get at – most likely the biscuits! Eat first.
- Make it a rule that you eat at the table. There isn't a short cut round this, but it helps to think of someone you admire, who has the figure you covet the most, and who you know eats correctly all the time. If she can do it, so can you.
- Put your knife and fork down every time you have put something into your mouth. Don't pick them up again until you've swallowed.
- Chew everything 15–20 times, whether you want to or not. You'll soon get into the swing of it!
- Make a decision that the whole family waits five minutes after the main course has been cleared before the next course. Again, this is tedious until you get used to it, but soon you'll wonder how on earth you used to manage to bolt your food!

## Improve Your General Health

So far, I've talked about the chaos of your hormones and the chaos of your mind, but one very important factor is your general health and stress level. You already know that stress causes the release of the hormones adrenalin and cortisol, and these rob your body of their defences allowing scavenging free radicals, which have been released because of the overwhelming attack on your body, to roam about causing damage and destruction. In their wake you also have the effects of adrenalin burnout. You can catch every bug going; you can also be susceptible if you exercise too much, meaning that you are constantly asking your muscles to be regenerating and repairing themselves ready for the next attack, and this stresses your already overstretched system. Your hormones will be going into overdrive, trying desperately to keep one step ahead of your cigarette smoke, late nights, exercise, missed meals or overload from binges, and you're heading for the doctor saying something's not quite right! So let's look at how food can be useful to you in more ways than one.

### Step One – Protect from Inside

When you choose vegetables and fruits look for colour. The deeper the colour the more anti-oxidants they contain. These should all be on your shopping list:

- carrots
- red grapes rather than green
- red wine
- red onions rather than white
- pink grapefruit rather than yellow
- the darkest green vegetables
- brazil nuts

- mango
- whole fruits rather than just juices

## Step Two – Protect From Outside

An ageing body isn't necessarily an old one. An old body can still be supple, strong, and healthy rather than dried out, stiff and weak. Here are some measures you will need to take to keep looking good:

- Wear a hat or scarf whenever possible, especially in wind – don't worry about flattening your hair, your hair is ruined anyway if you keep stripping it of its oils with constantly gritty, fume-filled winds ripping through it. The sun does as much damage too. This way you can whip off your hat to reveal soft, conditioned tresses.
- Wear a high sun-protection factor face cream even on cloudy days. It's the light that causes the damage, not just the sun.
- Keep your joints mobilized every day. Your shoulder is capable of moving in a complete circle, your knee can fold back on itself. When did you last do these movements? Being stiff, looking bent or awkward or groaning with the effort when you reach or bend for something is reminiscent of an eighty-year-old, not a young woman of thirty. Being stiff is ageing, suppleness is youthful.

## Step Three – Protect Yourself From the Bugs!

Some people get everything going, others haven't had a cold or tummy bug for years, but experts believe that it is due to our failure of defence rather than overwhelming attack. As Dr Mike Hill, Chairman of the European Cancer Prevention Organisation says, 'I call it the garden-gate theory. I have a nice front garden which I have planted lovingly, spending a fortune on plants, tools and machinery, topped off with a garden gate and fencing. Then I leave the gate open, a dog comes in and digs up the lot. The cause of the destruction isn't an overwhelming, mob-handed attack, but my failure to shut the gate. A tiny lack of defence can cause havoc.

'On the other hand, overwhelming attack happens when the poisons are so severe that nobody can defend themselves against them, and I'm thinking of cigarette smoke, asbestos, or major pollutants. You can defend yourself against bugs or sunlight, but smoke and asbestos are carcinogens which are too overwhelming for normal dietary defences, so you have to avoid them at all costs. For normal dietary protection from standard free-radical attack, make green and yellow fruits and vegetables a major feature of your daily meals.'

So it's simple to fight back and keep your youthful good looks for as long as possible and always try to get your nutrients from food rather than rely on supplements. In one small vegetable there are literally thousands of micro-nutrients which all support each other, and you simply can't get all these from a supplement pill. Supplements are better than nothing, but they're a poor substitute for good food.

## Useful Microbes In Food

At birth, your gut is sterile. Bacteria are gradually acquired from your surroundings and you become colonized by microbes, the numbers of which change as you get older. Again, protection from attack is preferable to shutting the stable door afterwards with courses of antibiotics, because these can kill a lot of friendly gut flora and leave you with more problems. You need to resist colonization of the unfriendly bugs by operating a 'barrier-effect' – a carpet of micro-organisms which prevent attack by other unfriendly flora.

## Your best foods

- artichokes
- asparagus
- banana
- chicory
- leeks
- onions
- dairy products
- live yoghurt

These are your armoury!

## Your Plan of Action

1. Get more daylight. Light deprivation alters brain chemistry in many people, and makes them crave sugars and starches. These foods give a much-needed dose of the brain chemical serotonin, responsible for lifting mood and suppressing appetite. Lack of light causes carbohydrate cravings because in winter your body senses hibernation mode, and it stocks up on glucose. Get up earlier for an extra hour of daylight, put your desk near a window if possible, go for a walk outside at lunchtime – anything – but don't spend your days in artificial light. Daylight makes us more cheerful and positive. On the other hand, protect yourself from damaging ultra-violet light with sunscreens and hair protection.

2. Give your circulation a run every day. Shallow breathing means less oxygen gets to your blood and less blood flows to the capillaries. Allowing your blood to plod around day after day like sludge means your circulation isn't getting the workout it needs for supple arteries and healthy, pumping lungs. Good circulation also helps your

skin to avoid that 'slabby', thick look. A daily, twenty-minute circulation run will do more for you than almost anything else.

3. Start to exercise with weights. Your muscle is slowly beginning to diminish and this causes a slower metabolism. Muscles are live, they have a blood flow and a job to do, whereas fat does nothing. Keep muscles toned with twice-weekly workouts for upper and lower body. In the past, women didn't have to worry about toning as they got enough muscle work with day-to-day activities like carrying washing or buckets of coal. Start using weights when you're twenty-five, but if you've already gone past this don't worry. It is better to start late than not start at all.

4. Start to fight the oxidants or 'free radicals' which attack your immune system. See every day as another chance to hang on to your youthful looks by stopping your biological clock. Eat stir-fries with green and yellow peppers, nuts for vitamin E, add wheatgerm to your daily cereal or yoghurt, have tomatoes in sandwiches.

5. Eat regularly. You can get away (just) with erratic eating when you're a teenager, but many of the anguished letters about mood swings, fat thighs, misshapen abdomens and chronic tiredness come from women who just won't heed the warnings about regular eating. Your body needs regular meals!

6. Avoid surges in blood-sugar levels by eating moderate-sized meals. Large meals stimulate insulin surges and insulin stimulates the lipoprotein lipase, a hormone which promotes fat storage. Insulin response must be kept low.

7. Find your desirable weight and keep within 3kg either way. Constant weight swings are bad for your health.

8. Don't get sloppy. If you don't have anywhere to go and nobody more exciting to talk to than your three-year-old, it's tempting to wear the same old tracksuit bottoms and pull your hair up into a ponytail. This only makes you feel worse. At least wear some jeans or something which fits and makes you hold yourself in, otherwise you'll have no incentive to train those tummy muscles. Wear some make-up, otherwise you'll get depressed with yourself every time you look in a mirror. No time? Yes you have. It takes two and a half minutes to pat your face with foundation, slick on some lipstick and apply some mascara. It takes one and a half minutes to take it off again. Once you look better you'll be more likely to avoid the next biscuit or chocolate bar.

9. Find another way of dealing with stressful situations. How about a plain refusal, such as when asked to host a home-sales party for example, or go to a club with colleagues. Don't rustle through your diary and say you might be interested when the time comes, or go along and hate every moment. They will ring you another time, so this is delaying the stress. Simply say with a bright smile, 'Oh, no. It's not my sort of thing at all!' And leave them in no doubt that the subject is closed. You can do it, and always think – this is YOUR health at stake!!

# Chapter Nine

# So What do I Have to Eat?

This section is all about the different types of diet you can try in your battle against body chaos. I have taken a great deal of advice on each diet, not just from the experts but from the people who matter most – the women who have achieved success with them. There is a basic weight-loss diet, a PMS diet, a menopause diet, a wheat-free diet and more. I think that you will find something to suit you, but the big question is: do these diets work?

A diet doesn't work. Just like a car doesn't work on its own, a diet needs you if it's going to be effective. Just think – if someone could come up with a diet which worked by itself, weight problems would be a thing of the past, and someone would be very, very rich! All I can ever hope to do is to bring order into your eating chaos, and make suggestions which, if followed to the letter, will achieve weight loss through calorie deficit, give you all the nutrients you need, and be reasonably easy and enjoyable to be on.

Haven't you ever noticed that nobody ever ponders over what they are going to have for breakfast – or for lunch, for that matter? We don't study an array of cereals, breads, bacons and fruits and ask the family what they'd like for a change. We only get hung up about our evening meal, and many a food manufacturer's fortune has been made on the back of our need to enjoy this one meal of the day, and have some variety. Indeed, it tends not to be our entire day's food intake that worries us so much as the food we eat in the evening. Sitting down, relaxing, having time on our hands and dare I say it – boredom – are the reasons that most of us consume much more than half our daily calories at this one meal – and this at a time when we are winding down and thinking of sleep! So the first decision you have to make is to get rid of those blips on your meal graph and even out the size and frequency of your meals.

Looking at what I have just said, you can see that you aren't going to have to worry about planning for lots and lots of complicated meals every week – in fact just seven! You can forget about breakfast, and lunch can be one of a small list of favourites, so you only need worry about seven meals a week. And please do think in terms of meals. In my mailbag each week I sift through hundreds of letters, all saying, 'These are the foods I like . . . these are the foods I hate.' But you don't eat mince or pasta or onions, you eat shepherd's pie, spaghetti bolognese, scrambled eggs on toast. So always draw up a shortlist of the meals you like, and write your shopping list from these.

Personally, I never touch convenience foods. You mustn't hide behind the excuse of being too busy to cook, because you don't need to cook. Salads are easy, an omelette is easier still and a jacket potato is easiest of all. People overestimate the length of time it takes to prepare meals properly, but the other factor in the equation is that you tend to eat convenience meals which you wouldn't have bothered to make, such as macaroni cheese or lasagne. I mean, would you fiddle about with all that cheese sauce? Me neither, and that's why you'd stay slimmer and healthier without it.

# The BEAT YOUR BODY CHAOS Diet

### Turn back the clock in 28 days!

This is a basic, calorie-restricted diet, which will also help to control cravings and banish binges – the twin curses of hormonal hell. If your body chaos is caused or exacerbated by excess weight, this diet will help you to lose over 6 kilos in six weeks, or 4.5 to 5.5 kilos by the end of the month. And you'll do it safely. You will need to continue this regime over a period of months to really see the long-term benefits of sensible dieting, so get the hang of it so you can adapt it to your own schedule.

## Planning a Weight-loss Diet

I am going to give you not just a diet, but an eating plan that *works* – after all eating can be a pleasure or a mundane ritual or simply a physical necessity, but if you have a weight problem that bothers you, food is a threat. This diet is going to be very simple, therefore, because surrounding yourself with the enemy seems to be how just about every diet starts off: you decide to eat less, so you go to the shops armed with a longer shopping list than usual; you work out that cooking is the temptation yet you're scouring low-fat cookery books. OK, you can't avoid eating, but you can avoid rubbing salt into the dieting wound by mixing and grating and steaming a lot of things you can only eat half of!

When on a weight-loss diet, the purpose is to reduce calories without reducing nutrients. Planning a weight-loss diet simply needs an energy reduction of 500-800 calories a day, so the easiest and most sensible way to start is to cut out all the food and drink which supply the most useless calories – so-called 'empty' calories – which have almost no nutritional good points. The first things that spring to mind are alcohol and sugar.

Alcohol is not banned on this diet, but you must get a grip on drink that is a pleasant accompaniment to a meal, or a drink that you are having simply because there's a good film on, or because you want to stay up that bit later, or simply to finish the bottle. If you want a drink at these times, have some juice, mineral water or tea.

## The Rules

### Rule 1: start strong – eat within an hour of waking

Your systems have started cranking into action, and blood-sugar levels are low. You might argue that you have no time for eating, but this could be the key to your weight problem. Eating at this time prevents over-eating later.

### Rule 2: lunch must be substantial

'Substantial' does not mean a lot, but it does mean what it says. This time of day is the start of the long haul when you have several hours' work left, then you have to travel home or need to start other tasks once you get home, so you need a meal of some substance, not just a yoghurt and an apple! Although the lunches I have suggested are mainly spiced rice with sultanas and some fruit, they still have enough good-quality calories to see you through a long afternoon. This is NOT the meal which is used to save calories for weight loss.

## Rule 3: eat light in the evening

This probably goes against everything you have been doing for years, but you simply don't need the sort of food that gives you bursts of energy in the evening, when all you are going to do is sit and relax. You have probably been eating two-thirds of your daily calories in this one meal alone, which is just not commonsense. You can still have a nice plate of something which is sociable – not just a bite of toast and a few beans! – but the calories must be light.

The only exception to this rule is after a good-quality exercise session (not just a gentle stroll round the block), in which case you need to re-fuel your muscles within an hour and a half.

## What If You Get Hungry?

You are on a diet, and it is important to try and train your appetite. However, if you find it unbearable you can either:

- Drink a glass of skimmed milk.
- Make a cup or mug of hot milk sweetened with sugar.
- Make a hot milky coffee and have with an apple.
- Have a pot of spiced rice (see page 288).

## The Secrets

### Milk

The base of this diet is milk, and you may drink as much skimmed or semi-skimmed milk as you like at any time you feel hungry. If you do not like milk, the soya alternative called 'So Good' is probably the best-tasting drink I have had, and I swap between the dairy and non-dairy variety regularly. Both cow's milk and soya milk are excellent for providing a range of vitamins, minerals and protein, plus essential carbohydrates for energy. Indeed, milk is often quite rightly called a 'food'.

Milk-based desserts are also a feature of this diet, especially my creamy spiced rice (see page 288). Again, I have specifically created this easy meal to be made in advance, in quantity, so it is ready and available whenever you need it. With its rice, dried fruit and milk, you will have instant long-lasting energy and, of course, the nutrition and calming effects that can only come from the enzymes in milk.

## Apricot and Almond Crunch

This is an invention of mine which I called 'The Crunch' and is a simple meal of cereals, dried fruits, nuts and seeds which is similar to some commercial muesli products, but different in that I have always eaten this as a meal at any time. The beauty is in the simplicity. It contains some of the most important nutrients you will ever need, right there in a little container you can tote around with you, so simple it is even more convenient than those little pots of savoury noodles you just add boiling water to. You just add milk and maybe a sliced apple, a few grapes or other fruit, or maybe even a spoonful of yoghurt. It is a complete meal in a pot, and you can make enough for the whole week in about three minutes.

## Basic 'Crunch' bowl

Forget weighing and measuring – for this diet you only need a standard-sized teacup for all your ingredients.

| | |
|---|---|
| 2 cups plain oats | 1 cup sunflower seeds |
| 2 cups Grape Nuts (purchased cereal) | 1 cup flaked almonds |
| 1 cup wheat germ (Froment or Bemax are best) | 1 cup large sultanas and raisins mixed |
| | 1 cup dried apricots, chopped finely |

Mix together, and keep in a snap-shut container. This quantity makes 9 portions. For a portion, simply scoop out a teacupful and add a full teacup of cold skimmed milk. Top with half a banana, sliced, and 1 tbsp natural organic yoghurt.

This Crunch meal has everything you could want for health and beauty:

- Apricots: iron, zinc, carbohydrates, potassium, fibre, extremely low in saturated fat.
- Oats: soluble fibre, protein, very low in saturated fat.
- Grape Nuts: protein, niacin, extremely low in saturated fat.
- Raisins: natural sugars, fibre.
- Sunflower seeds: high polyunsaturated fats, vitamin B1, iron, protein, niacin, fibre.
- Almonds: high protein, copper, vitamins B, E, iron, zinc, fibre, mono-unsaturated fats, fibre. Very low in saturated fat.

## Drinks

Drink plain mineral or tap water which is flavoured with slices of fresh orange, and have this at every meal as well as in-between meals. Fruit and herbal teas are also recommended.

## Protein Vitality Drink

| | |
|---|---|
| 1 banana | 150 ml skimmed milk |
| 1 medium carton plain bio yoghurt | |

Blend all three ingredients together in a food processor or blender for 20 seconds until smooth. Drink as soon as possible, but do not hurry it!

## WEEK ONE

### Monday

Breakfast

One portion Crunch topped with half a banana, sliced and 1 teacupful skimmed milk (must be skimmed). Portion of grapefruit and orange segments, mixed. (I suggest you buy tinned – often called 'Florida cocktail' or something similar. Or you can make your own, by preparing plenty in advance and keeping refrigerated for the week.)

Mid-morning

Portion creamy spiced rice (see page 288). One apple.

Lunch

Portion main meal salad (see page 284), slice apricot and almond flapjack (see page 274). One pear.

Main Meal

175g chicken or Quorn pieces, stir-fried with plenty of mixed colourful vegetables and a dash of soy sauce. Fresh fruit salad.

### Tuesday

Breakfast

Crunch cereal with a quarter of an apple, sliced. Glass fresh orange juice.

Mid-morning

Apple, milky coffee or glass of skimmed milk.

Lunch

Protein vitality drink, slice apricot and almond flapjack (see page 274), small bunch grapes.

Main Meal

Two-egg omelette with herbs, mixed salad with a little

French dressing made with walnut oil. Three different green vegetables, one of which should be starchy, such as peas or broad beans.

## Wednesday

### Breakfast
Portion of porridge made thus: 40g rolled oats and 1 tbsp medium oatmeal mixed with 200ml water. Microwave or simmer for 2–3 minutes, leave to cool and add as much skimmed milk or soya milk as you like and either 1 tsp sugar OR golden syrup. Two tbsp grapefruit segments.

### Mid-morning
Protein vitality drink. Few grapes.

### Lunch
Two Ryvitas topped with a sliced hard-boiled egg. Portion spiced rice (see page 288). Apple.

### Main Meal
Swedish Cod: fry one large thinly sliced potato in vegetable oil, when virtually cooked add a fillet of cod to the pan. Serve on a bed of 3 tablespoons mixed sweet corn and peas. Cook 1 portion potatoes extra, and leave cold. Bowl mixed berries (strawberries, blueberries, raspberries) with 1 tbsp natural yoghurt.

## Thursday

### Breakfast
Portion Crunch with 10 halved grapes.

### Mid-morning
Milky drink or milkshake. Apple.

### Lunch
28g piece of cheese, sliced on to a crispbread. Pot creamy spiced rice (see page 288).

## Main Meal

Large fillet or sirloin steak, grilled tomato and mushrooms, peas and mixed salad. Fruit yoghurt (see page 280) OR banana and tofu cream dessert (see page 277).

## Friday

### Breakfast

Portion porridge made as for the recipe given on Wednesday and usual portion skimmed milk. Glass fresh orange juice.

### Mid-morning

Protein vitality drink. Apple.

### Lunch

Colourful mixed salad sandwich on granary or wholemeal bread, including watercress and red peppers. Portion fresh fruit salad.

### Main Meal

Skinless, boneless chicken breast, marinated in lemon juice with a few coriander leaves, grilled or pan-fried and served on a bed of mixed peas and broad beans OR spinach. Vegetarian alternative: Use Quorn cubes, adding 1 dsp cashew nuts. Stewed apple or rhubarb served on top of 2 tbsp plain yoghurt.

## Saturday

### Breakfast

Portion Crunch topped with sliced mango.

### Mid-morning

Milky coffee or milkshake. Piece fruit.

### Lunch

Small container or plateful of carrot and celery sticks, with some cauliflower florets, and a little cottage or half-fat cream cheese as a dip (about 1 tbsp). Bowl spiced rice (see page 288), surrounded by sliced banana and mango.

### Main Meal
Plain tuna fish salad, using 100g tuna, sweetcorn, mixed red and yellow peppers and a few cold, cooked French beans. Fruit yoghurt (see page 280) OR banana and tofu cream dessert (see page 277).

## Sunday

### Breakfast
Bowl Crunch with yoghurt topping and 2 sliced tinned or fresh apricots. Portion of grapefruit and orange segments.

### Mid-morning
Protein vitality drink OR hot chocolate (use the low-calories sachets) made with skimmed milk. Small handful salted peanuts.

### Lunch
Portion main meal salad (see page 284), including ingredients you like, such as avocado, prawns or ham. A banana.

### Main Meal
Large jacket potato, filled with *either* 2 tbsp cottage cheese OR 2 tbsp tuna fish OR 60g grated hard cheese OR 1 tbsp bacon bits and a hard-boiled egg. Colourful mixed salad. Half packet crisps. Fresh fruit salad.

## WEEK TWO

### Monday

Breakfast, mid-morning and lunch
As first week.

## Main Meal

One portion chicken which has been marinated in orange juice (see page 281) (freshly-squeezed), and a little of the grated orange rind. Grill or shallow fry, then add to a bed of mixed vegetables of your choice. Vegetarian alternative: use Quorn cubes, marinate and use in the same way. Fresh fruit salad.

## Tuesday

### Breakfast, mid-morning and lunch

As first week.

### Main Meal

Two poached eggs with 3 rashers well-grilled bacon, grilled tomato and 2 tbsp baked beans. Vegetarian alternative: two-egg cheese or herb omelette filled with baked beans and served with salad. Yoghurt and stewed fruit.

## Wednesday

### Breakfast, mid-morning and lunch

As first week.

### Main Meal

Plain pan-fried or roasted fillet of salmon, served on a bed of mixed peas and sweetcorn with a dressing made from equal parts mayonnaise and half-fat crème fraiche, with some snipped fronds of dill. Bowl mixed berries (strawberries, blueberries, raspberries) with 1 tbsp natural yoghurt.

## Thursday

### Breakfast, mid-morning and lunch

As first week.

### Main Meal

*Either* fillet steak as for Thursday of Week One OR a pork steaklet and mixed steamed vegetables with a little gravy

*OR* a portion of beef bouguignonne (see page 277) served with broccoli and peas. Vegetarian alternative: main meal salad (see page 284) with avocado and prawns (if you eat shellfish). Fruit yoghurt (see page 280) OR banana and tofu cream dessert (see page 277).

## Friday

**Breakfast, mid-morning and lunch**
As first week.

**Main Meal**
Stir-fried vegetable curry (see page 288) OR chilli (see page 291), made with mixed beans and vegetables, in a very low-fat sauce. (This means that only tomatoes and chilli powder have been added, no oils or fats.) No rice with this, it is served on a bed of grated raw vegetables such as carrot and white cabbage. Portion fresh fruit salad.

## Saturday

**Breakfast, mid-morning and lunch**
As first week.

**Main Meal**
Spaghetti Bolognese. Traditional Bolognese or vegetable sauce made with tinned tomatoes and extra lean mince. Serve on 90g (dry weight) spaghetti, no more, and have a colourful mixed salad to go with it. Bowl of mixed berries or fresh strawberries, topped with yoghurt.

## Sunday

**Breakfast, mid-morning and lunch**
As first week.

**Main Meal**
Large potato, (about 200–250g) boiled and mashed, served

with 3 slices lean ham and 2 sliced tomatoes OR mixed cooked vegetables topped with 60g hard cheese, grated. Half packet salted peanuts. Fresh fruit salad.

## WEEK THREE

### Monday
Breakfast, mid-morning and lunch
As first week.

### Main Meal
Chicken stir-fry with mixed colourful vegetables OR chicken curry portion (should be chicken tikka or similar, which is 'dry fried'. Quorn cubes or tofu can be used as a vegetarian alternative. Fresh fruit salad.

### Tuesday

Breakfast, mid-morning and lunch
As first week.

### Main Meal
Small slice (quarter of the whole) broccoli and Stilton quiche, served with colourful mixed salad. Fresh fruit salad.

### Wednesday

Breakfast, mid-morning and lunch
As first week.

### Main Meal
Smoked salmon salad: two slices smoked salmon, half avocado sliced, 1 tbsp fresh prawns, served on a bed of salad OR plain cod fillet, baked in milk then topped with parsley, served with mashed carrots, mashed broccoli and peas.

Bowl mixed berries (strawberries, blueberries, raspberries) with 1 tbsp natural yoghurt.

## Thursday

### Breakfast, mid-morning and lunch
As first week.

### Main Meal
Steak in pepper sauce – pan-fry and before serving add 2 tbsp brandy, 1 tbsp half-fat crème fraiche and 1 tsp steak pepper or freshly-milled black peppercorns. Serve on bed of 2 tbsp rice with 2 green vegetables. Vegetarian alternative: vegetables in a pepper sauce made as above, should include pulses and extra pine kernels or nuts. Have one extra tbsp rice. Stewed fruit with 2 tbsp plain fromage frais.

## Friday

### Breakfast, mid-morning and lunch
As first week.

### Main Meal
Small pizza topped with either chillies and spiced beef or chilli mixed vegetables. Side salad, which must include red peppers and watercress. Sliced fresh pineapple with a dipping sauce made from a few fresh strawberries (tinned will do). Simply process the strawberries for a few seconds until they make a runny sauce.

## Saturday

### Breakfast, mid-morning and lunch
As first week.

### Main Meal
Pork or lamb chop or steaklet, simply grilled and served with steamed or boiled broccoli, carrots and cauliflower, no

potatoes. Vegetarian alternative: mixed vegetable lasagne. Cook the vegetables as above, cover with a simple, very low-fat white sauce made from skimmed milk and cornflour. Boil one teacup (dried weight) of pasta shapes, drain and cool. Add 3 rashers chopped grilled bacon or 2 slices ham, chopped, a handful of fresh spinach leaves and 1 tbsp half-fat crème fraiche. Add a little garlic (optional), chopped parsley and serve with a side salad of sliced tomatoes in olive oil.

Vegetarian alternative: use spinach, broad beans and peas, and add fresh coriander leaves, half-fat crème fraiche and garlic.

Fresh fruit salad.

## Sunday

### Breakfast, mid-morning and lunch
As first week.

### Main Meal
Three small roast potatoes with either roast chicken, beef or other meat of your choice. Three vegetables, lightly boiled. Gravy and stuffing where appropriate. Vegetarian alternative: breaded Quorn portion with roast potatoes and vegetables as above. Fresh fruit salad. Small slice sponge cake OR 3 chocolate digestive biscuits.

## WEEK FOUR

### Monday

### Breakfast, mid-morning and lunch
As first week.

### Main Meal
Fillet of smoked haddock or cod, poached in milk, served

with peas and sweetcorn. Sweet Marscapone mousse (see page 289).

## Tuesday

Breakfast, mid-morning and lunch
As first week.

Main Meal
Stuffed tomatoes: using four large tomatoes, stuff with 45g grated hard cheese such as Cheddar. Place on baking sheet and bake in hot oven for 5 minutes. Turn on the grill and put the tomatoes under it until brown on top. Serve on 2 slices bread which has been sprayed or brushed with a little olive oil, and grilled in the oven at the same time as the tomatoes. This makes lightly fried bread. Baked apple: core a large baking apple and fill with sultanas. Brush with butter and bake for 20–30 minutes in a medium oven. Serve with either 1 dsp custard or 1 dsp half-fat fromage frais.

## Wednesday

Breakfast, mid-morning and lunch
As first week.

Main Meal
Plain stir-fried chicken breast with mixed colourful vegetables and soy sauce. Stewed apple and yoghurt.

## Thursday

Breakfast, mid-morning and lunch
As first week.

Main Meal
Light meal of double quantity lentil soup (see page 282) (400ml) with one small wholemeal roll. Fresh fruit salad.

## Friday

Breakfast, mid-morning and lunch
As first week.

Main Meal
Vegetable or beef chilli served, not with rice, but on a bed of grated vegetables. Fresh fruit salad.

## Saturday

Breakfast, mid-morning and lunch
As first week.

Main Meal
Fillet or rump steak with mixed salad. Vegetarian alternative: main meal salad (see page 284). Winter fruit salad (see page 281) with a dsp fromage frais on top and a sprinkling of flaked almonds.

## Sunday

Breakfast, mid-morning and lunch
As first week.

Main Meal
Two slices roast beef or chicken with 3 different vegetables, including carrots. Apple and blackberries with custard OR bowl of mixed banana slices and 10 sliced grapes, topped with 1 dsp custard.


Well done!! You have finished the diet and should have lost weight, and learned a little about appetite control. Dieting is hard, but it *never* makes people fat, as some old stories tell you it does. This is a myth put about by people in whose best interests it is to 'knock' the weight-loss industry, but I have always found that by careful management of diet, a desirable weight and good figure are maintained for life, quite painlessly. It is the eating that makes people fat!

## Where Do I Go From Here?

You need to observe the general guidelines from the Body Chaos diet.

- Eat a substantial amount of calories at breakfast.
- Eat little and often.
- Do not make one meal much bigger than the others.
- Eat lightly in the evening.
- Drink milk.

## A Note About Weighing Yourself

Obviously you should weigh yourself once a week to keep tabs on how you are doing, but don't get hung up about it. Remember that your body has no idea what a week is: weeks and months are man-made units of time that we find useful, but your body only understands rhythms and fluctuations over day and night, winter and summer, months and years. If you have not lost much weight one week, it is only significant if this is a general trend and you lose no weight for weeks on end. If this is the case your energy balance is not right and you should either exercise more, or start to be careful about the exact amounts of food you are eating. *Whatever you do, don't get worked up about a weekly weigh-in!* – but be sure that the general trend is downwards.

# Water Retention Prevention Diet

Water retention is another nasty problem during the month, making you feel fat, unattractive and edgy. It is quite an easy problem to beat, so don't despair.

## Your Plan of Action

1. Watch the salt. While your body is designed to cope with excess salt, it does make tissues hold water and this is a factor if you have high blood pressure or are prone to water retention. Your body tends to hold water at certain times of the month anyway, so there is hardly any point in making matters worse. You should consume around 1,200mg a day of sodium, but we all run the risk of eating much larger amounts simply because manufacturers add it to our food. It is estimated that about 9g of salt is added to our daily food, which is 3,600g sodium – three times the amount you need. However at the time of writing there is a drive to introduce better ranges of low-salt or no-added salt ranges of food into our supermarkets. There are also many natural foods which are high in salt, so keep an eye on them until you get to be an expert on sodium.

2. Start by substituting low-sodium meals in the week before your period – it also doesn't hurt to adopt these practices and habits as much as possible ordinarily, limiting the high-salt alternatives for nights out and parties.

3. Be aware of high-salt traps:

   - Watch the beer – there's 25 mg sodium in approximately every quarter litre.
   - Be careful about home-water softeners: they add sodium to the water.
   - Steer clear of laxatives – most contain sodium.
   - Watch out for diet sodas – the calories might be low but the sodium is high!

4. Balance out with potassium. Even if your latest meal was high in salt don't panic. Potassium regulates sodium, but many diets are so poor that they don't have enough potassium to beat the damage. Make sure you have plenty of high-potassium foods in your diet such as: bananas, chicken, apricots, potatoes, chickpeas, milk, red meat, fish.

5. Eat as many diuretic foods as possible. Naturally diuretic foods include: celery, parsley, strawberries, asparagus.

6. Drink 2.25 litres plain water every day. Yes, strange though it may sound, drinking extra water actually stops you retaining water. It makes sense, because your body will only ever hold a certain amount, so you will never feel 'waterlogged' – just fresher and without stale fluids hanging around in your body – flush 'em out!!

## Your Sample Diet for Beating Water Retention

This is a low-sodium diet to stop excess fluid building up in your tissues. Keep to this diet, or a variation, if you suffer from high blood pressure, and use it for two weeks before your period if you suffer monthly fluid retention that resolves itself when your period starts.

### Foods you must avoid

- all foods in brine – e.g. tuna, tinned vegetables
- baked beans, crisps, salted nuts

- preserved meats e.g. ham, bacon, pork pies, pates
- tinned salmon, shrimps, cockles
- cheese
- salted butter
- crackers, cakes, most breads
- Bovril, Oxo, Marmite
- packet or tinned soups
- sweets and toffees

## Foods you should eat

Including food high in potassium which helps to balance fluid levels:

- fresh vegetables
- sodium-free bread
- muesli, Shredded Wheat, All Bran
- apricots, bananas
- potatoes
- pineapple
- tomatoes
- citrus fruit
- parsley
- asparagus and celery which are diuretic vegetables

## Energy Breaks – choose two a day

- fresh fruit salad
- banana sandwich with low-fat crème fraiche spread
- two Ryvita spread with sugar-free fruit spread
- apricot and almond flapjack (see page 274)
- slice carrot and orange cake (see page 278)
- slice date and walnut cake (see page 279)
- slice banana cake (see page 276)
- three water biscuits topped with sugar-free spread
- mixed raw vegetables e.g. carrot sticks, cauliflower florets

## Sample Seven-day Menu

### Day 1

Breakfast
Glass of fresh orange or grapefruit juice.
Rice Krispies with 150ml semi-skimmed milk.

Lunch
Avocado and 113g fresh prawns on salad greens. French bread. Mixed fruit in jelly.

Main Meal
Plain cod fillet, baked in milk which is then thickened to a simple parsley sauce (using cornflour, milk and fresh parsley, no butter), served on bed of carrot and swede puree, peas. Baked banana served with 1 tbsp crème fraiche.

### Day 2

Breakfast
Glass of fresh pineapple juice. Bowl plain porridge, 150ml semi-skimmed milk, 1 tsp sugar.

Lunch
Bowl celery or asparagus soup with low-salt bread slices. Pineapple and mango chunks in plain fromage frais.

Main Meal
Stir-fried chicken strips in curry spices and 1 tbsp oil, served on plain Basmati rice which has been boiled and then fried in the chicken juices. Side salad of lamb's lettuce, celery, mango, sliced tomato and cucumber. Meringue filled with fresh fruit, served with 1 tbsp single cream.

## Day 3

### Breakfast
Glass of fresh orange or grapefruit juice. Rice Krispies with semi-skimmed milk.

### Lunch
Avocado and 113g fresh prawns on salad greens, top with a few cold asparagus spears, French bread. Mixed fruit in jelly.

### Main Meal
Plain fillet steak, grilled, served on a bed of steamed spinach with a sauce made from crushed black peppercorns and 1 tbsp half-fat crème fraiche, stirred into the pan juices. Plain yoghurt with 6 dried, chopped apricots.

## Day 4

### Breakfast
Glass of fresh orange or grapefruit juice. Plain porridge with 150ml warm skimmed milk, 1 tsp sugar, 1 dsp Froment.

### Lunch
Ciabatta loaf topped with tomato, onion and pepper mixture (tinned is best), little olive oil drizzled over, grilled, then topped with 1 tsp Parmesan cheese. Two celery sticks. Apple.

### Main Meal
Slice of salmon and broccoli flan, generous serving colourful mixed salad. Winter fruit salad (see page 281) served with a little single cream or custard.

## Day 5

### Breakfast
Two eggs, poached, on two slices granary bread, OR tomatoes on toast, no salt.

**Lunch**
Main meal salad (see page 284), one slice sundried tomato or herb bread. Banana and a few dried apricots.

**Main Meal**
Grilled salmon or cod fillet, plain mashed potatoes, 3 tbsp carrots, steamed asparagus spears, parsley. Hot grilled pineapple pieces, with 1 dsp crème fraiche.

## Day 6

**Breakfast**
Bowl of fresh fruit salad, including melon. Two Shredded Wheat, 1 tsp sugar, 200ml skimmed milk.

**Lunch**
Three slices cold chicken, 2 tomatoes, sliced, 2 pieces French bread, 3 celery sticks. Banana sliced into plain fromage frais and topped with 2 tsp Froment.

**Main Meal**
Stir-fried vegetable curry (see page 288) OR chicken and vegetable stir-fry curry OR plain lamb chop, grilled, with cauliflower and broad beans and boiled potatoes. Winter fruit salad (see page 286) and fromage or crème fraiche.

## Day 7

**Breakfast**
Glass of fresh orange or grapefruit juice. Rice Krispies with semi-skimmed milk.

**Lunch**
Celery or asparagus soup, 2 slices wholemeal bread with unsalted butter. Gooseberry fool (see page 286).

**Main Meal**
Spaghetti bolognese with a colourful mixed salad. Banana

and pineapple pieces, mixed in a fruit salad topped with a sprinkling of flaked almonds.

## Sensible Wheat-free Diet

### Bloating

There can't be a woman alive who hasn't suffered from uncomfortable bloating from time to time. Most women suffer all the time. It's that feeling that you just can't hold in your tummy however hard you try and however empty your stomach is. But don't let this particular chaos ruin your life. Food can be the trigger, but an even more significant cause of bloating is not eating. Leaving long gaps between meals, skipping meals because you're rushed off your feet and eating too quickly, neither pausing for breath nor chewing food thoroughly – these are even more likely causes of bloating.

It's not so much what you eat but how and when you eat. You don't stop eating certain foods but you eat them at a different time of the day from when you might normally have them. You cut out certain chemicals and natural foods known to cause wind, and you get a grip on constipation. In five days a miraculous transformation takes place and your stomach is suddenly flatter and in control. The added benefit of this quick-fix is purely psychological, but I'm all for that. Feeling slimmer makes you act slimmer, makes you stand taller and tighten your belt a notch or two. Confidence is your greatest ally in the war against body chaos, so if you are a martyr to bloating, follow these simple rules:

- Don't eat any fruit before 7 p.m.
- Only eat soluble fibre for breakfast, e.g. porridge oats, oat-based muesli, Rice Krispies, Special K.
- Chew everything slowly and don't swallow until your food feels mushy in your mouth.
- Don't chew gum – you swallow a lot of air.
- Don't have bran, strawberries or nuts before 7 p.m.
- Don't have onions, pulses, broccoli, cauliflower, cabbage, asparagus, leeks – at least until the evening.
- No 'diet' mousses or yoghurts which contain artificial sweetener, carageenan, Xanthan Gum or Guar Gum.
- Do have a bowl of All-Bran or Weetabix in the evening topped with mixed fruit salad with banana.
- Do have natural 'live' bio yoghurt with stewed fruit and a topping of nuts or seeds later in the day.
- Drink plain water with all meals.

## Hormonal Bloating

Bloating can also be a side-effect of the time of the month, when you might not be retaining fluids, but you feel as if you are. Weight gain at this time is probable, but my research shows that it is more likely that you are eating slightly more because you are feeling so lousy! I don't need to tell you how dreadful it feels to have your clothes just that bit too tight and your stomach just a little bit too hot and gassy and tight, but I have found that it is what you do as a result which causes the most problems. If you feel fat and unattractive, you're more likely to throw caution to the winds and binge on food, and this is the reason you gain weight. Like all weight gain during the time of the month, it goes quickly enough when your hormones get back to square one.

## Your Plan of Action

1. Follow the advice above for no more than five days out of seven when bloating is a problem.

2. Do five minutes of abdominal exercises, followed by a full five minutes of stretches for your midsection. This will create a feeling of firmness and control.

3. Go for a walk or, even better, do forty-five minutes of hard cardiovascular exercise – something which makes you really pour with sweat.

4. Don't wear clothing which is too loose however bloated you might feel. It leads to sloppiness and not bothering to hold yourself properly.

5. Don't miss meals – an empty stomach is more likely to lead to wind and bloating than a nicely full one.

6. Don't eat any meal from a plate bigger than a side plate. If necessary, divide your meal into two portions and eat them two hours apart. This also gives you something else to look forward to.

7. Watch your posture. Bad posture will add another few inches to your stomach area, you will catch sight of yourself and this will escalate to negative thoughts.

## Could It Be Wheat?

Some people blame bloating on a sensitivity to wheat. I have always been sceptical, but it's true that we have so much more wheat in our diets these days than we used to, and like anything which you eat too much, it can cause our systems to complain at the work they're having to do. Wheat sensitivity is a condition which rarely lasts, so you don't have to steer clear of your favourite biscuits or cereals for ever. This is the myth. Once people have locked on to the fact that they might be sensitive to wheat, they worry that they're going to have to be a food detective for the rest of their lives, but in fact wheat sensitivity is usually a sign of your general nutritional status. Wheat is in everything! Not just biscuits, bread, cakes and pasta, but in sauces and mixes and spreads. You'll usually find that after a few wheat-free weeks you can start to re-introduce a few favourites one-by-one, and your problem will be sorted. It's also a good exercise in seeing what you can do without, and getting some routine into your meals. After all, you need that bread for your sandwiches and breakfast toast, but do you really need the two custard creams you have every day at coffee time? Don't answer that one!

## Diet

Follow this diet, making variations along the way to suit your personal preferences, for about four weeks. Gradually introduce your own favourites one a day after that, starting with a little cereal or toast.

### Energy breaks – choose no more than two a day

- coconut pyramid
- meringue
- macaroon
- oatcakes with cream cheese
- rice cakes with lemon curd or jam
- fresh fruit salad
- any piece fruit
- small pot rice pudding (see page 288)
- plain or fruit yoghurt (see page 280)

Do be aware of food content and eat accordingly, although if Irritable Bowel Syndrome (IBS) is suspected you might want to look at meal size and frequency of eating, along with meal content. For example, a large meal eaten after a long period of hunger will almost always cause gasiness, distended stomach and discomfort, whatever the food.

## Food you must avoid

- wheat germ
- wheat germ oil
- pancakes
- pizzas
- pitta bread
- chapattis
- biscuits
- pastry
- pasta
- scones
- crispbreads
- pies, wafers, cones
- gravy and sauces
- stuffing
- meat or fish in batter or breadcrumbs
- any food made with breadcrumbs

## Foods you should eat

- bacon
- butter and cheese
- coffee
- crisps
- dried fruit
- eggs
- fish and shellfish
- jams, honey
- milk
- oils

- meat, pork and poultry
- vegetables
- nuts and seeds
- rice, tapioca
- Marmite
- dried beans and pulses
- oatcakes and rice cakes

## Sample Seven-day Menu

### Day 1

**Breakfast**
40g Rice Krispies, 200ml semi-skimmed milk. Small bowl fresh fruit salad.

**Lunch**
Potato salad with strips of either smoked salmon or chicken. Small pot (150g) fruit yoghurt (see page 281).

**Main Meal**
Vegetable paella OR herb omelette with salad and a jacket potato. Meringue with fresh fruits.

### Day 2

**Breakfast**
40g oat-based muesli, topped with dried fruit and flaked almonds. 200ml glass of fresh orange juice.

**Lunch**
Tuna and rice salad OR hard-boiled egg salad. Apple and banana slices in fruit jelly.

**Main Meal**
Beef bourguignonne (see page 277) with mashed potatoes and fresh greens. Rice pudding (see page 288) with stewed fruit compote topping.

### Day 3

**Breakfast**
Half grapefruit. Two poached eggs, 2 rashers bacon, mushrooms, grilled tomatoes. Wheat-free toast and olive oil spread.

**Lunch**
Cottage cheese and fruit salad OR cottage cheese as a dip, sticks of carrot and celery, small packet crisps.

**Main Meal**
Small grilled fillet steak with a crème fraiche and pepper sauce, full salad, small portion sauté or boiled potatoes OR courgette and tomato gratin, side salad. Fresh fruit salad with portion ice cream.

### Day 4

**Breakfast**
40g Rice Krispies, 200ml milk, small bowl fresh fruit salad.

**Lunch**
Couscous with grilled vegetables OR 42g sliced cheese on 2–3 oatcakes, small bunch grapes. Apricot and almond flapjack (see page 274). Glass of fresh apple or orange juice.

**Main Meal**
Chicken and vegetable stir-fry with soy sauce OR baked/grilled chicken in orange marinade (see page 281), served with jacket potato and watercress. Winter fruit salad (see page 281) OR yoghurt with apricot and fig compote.

### Day 5

**Breakfast**
Bowl of citrus salad. Two slices of rye toast, marmalade.

**Lunch**
Jacket potato filled with tuna and peas. Garnish of green

salad leaves. Small pot fruit yoghurt (see page 280) topped with flaked nuts.

### Main Meal
Fillet of salmon, grilled or poached, served on a bed of mixed rice, peas and peppers, topped with a little dill mayonnaise. Meringue with fresh fruits.

## Day 6

### Breakfast
40g porridge made with 150ml milk. Small bowl citrus salad.

### Lunch
Chicken or egg sandwich on wheat-free bread. Banana and tofu cream dessert (see page 277) OR cream caramel.

### Main Meal
Beef bourguignonne (see page 277) from Day 2 with carrots and broccoli, boiled potatoes. Fresh fruit salad with cream or ice cream.

## Day 7

### Breakfast
Grapefruit segments. 40g oat-based muesli with 1 tsp Froment and 200ml milk.

### Lunch
Avocado and prawn salad on bed of mixed leaves, pine nuts on top, 1 dsp French dressing. Small pot chocolate mousse, few grapes.

### Main Meal
Shepherd's pie, cabbage, peas OR vegetable chilli (see page 291). Stewed fruit and custard OR meringue with fresh fruits.

# Good Mood Diet – Anti-stress, Anxiety and Depression

## Tired, Stressed, Anxious

There's nothing quite like anxiety and stress for wearing out your hormones. Insulin goes into overtime as you eat for comfort, have high sugar levels and take too little rest. If you are also getting up in the night to a baby or a dependent relative, you are ignoring your body clock by staying awake and being woken when your body wants to sleep. You can't wear out your melatonin, but by swimming against the tide all the time you'll simply increase the stress on your hormones.

This diet is amazing. It really works to calm your nerves slowly, wake you up from debilitating tiredness and help you look on the bright side. It works by stabilizing your blood-sugar levels, supplying B vitamins which are essential for nerves, and most important of all, stimulating the pathways to your brain chemical serotonin, the so-called 'happy hormone' which is made possible by the amino acid tryptophan. Tryptophan acts as a non-drug anti-depressant, it helps you sleep and reduces your sensitivity to pain, so you really can't lose. There are some wonderful foods around which actually do the same job as prescription tranquillizers. Your diet contains a plentiful amount, so try to ignore the fact that they might not be your cup of tea, and have them anyway, for example warm milk. Whenever I feel a difficult time ahead I rush to the microwave and warm a mug of milk, to which I add a teaspoon of sugar. Sugar is important, because it releases the right chemicals in the milk, so don't ignore it. Don't use artificial sweeteners either: they won't work.

It is also important to have plenty of the B vitamins when you are feeling stressed. They are particularly good for the nervous system, and are found in wheatgerm, meat, peas, potatoes, milk, eggs and pulses, among others.

### Energy breaks – two or three a day

Make sure you eat a light meal two hours before bed. Some ideas:

- small bowl lentil soup (see page 282)
- small bowl porridge
- slice of apricot and brazil nut bread (see page 275)
- Two Ryvitas with cottage cheese
- cottage cheese and celery or carrot sticks
- cup of warm skimmed milk with 1 tsp sugar

### Foods you should avoid

- caffeine – in coffee, chocolate and tea
- alcohol
- sweets and sugary snacks

### Basic preparations

1. Topping Mix: into an airtight container, empty one packet each of sunflower seeds, pumpkin seeds, sesame seeds, a small packet flaked almonds, 3 tbsp sultanas and 10 brazil nuts, flaked or chopped roughly. Keep in a cool place.

2. Make a half litre rice pudding according to recipe on page 288.

3. Make a citrus fruit salad from orange and grapefruit segments in natural juice, mixed with 2 tbsp raisins. Keep refrigerated.

## Sample Seven-day Menu

### Day 1

**Breakfast**
Grapefruit or 3 tbsp unsweetened grapefruit segments. Porridge with 1 dsp Froment, cup warm milk, tsp sugar. Tea or decaffeinated coffee.

**Lunch**
Avocado pear, sliced, 56g prawns, 2 tsp mayonnaise and tomato puree mixed on a bed of lettuce. Small pot natural fromage frais with sliced apple.

**Main Meal**
Thai turkey salad (see page 290). Winter fruit salad (see page 281) with crème fraiche.

### Day 2

**Breakfast**
2 tbsp citrus fruit salad. 3 tbsp home-made muesli or Familia topped with 1 tbsp topping mix, 200ml semi-skimmed milk.

**Lunch**
Jacket potato filled with 3 tbsp cottage cheese side salad of mixed peppers and celery. Sliced banana and apple mixed.

**Main Meal**
Meatballs in tomato sauce (see page 284) and mashed potatoes. Plain rice pudding with stewed apple.

### Day 3

**Breakfast**
40g porridge as Day 1. Banana.

**Lunch**
Cottage cheese and fruit salad.

**Main Meal**
Stir-fried chicken strips, topped with tomato and basil sauce (tinned), served on pasta shapes. Banana and custard.

## Day 4

**Breakfast**
Two Weetabix with hot milk, tsp sugar topped with 1 dsp Froment or natural wheatgerm, 10 grapes.

**Lunch**
2 tbsp tuna fish with potato salad and 2 tbsp sweetcorn. Slice carrot and orange cake (see page 278) and apple.

**Main Meal**
Salmon steak or fillet, grilled or poached, 4 tbsp brown rice, peas, cabbage, 2 boiled potatoes. Winter fruit salad (see page 281) topped with topping mix.

## Day 5

**Breakfast**
Citrus salad. 2 boiled eggs, 2 slices wholemeal toast OR All Bran with 150ml semi-skimmed or skimmed milk.

**Lunch**
Lentil or vegetable soup, granary or wholemeal roll. Small pot rice pudding (see page 288).

**Main Meal**
Liver with Dubonnet and orange (see page 283) on bed of mashed potatoes OR stir-fried tofu with mixed peppers on rice. Stewed fruit OR raspberry tofu whip.

## Day 6

### Breakfast
Porridge with 1 dsp Froment, cup of warm milk, 1 tsp sugar.
One slice granary toast with fruit spread.

### Lunch
Egg or beef sandwich on wholemeal with horseradish or
mayonnaise, lettuce. Slice apricot and almond flapjack (see
page 274).

### Main Meal
Roast beef, cabbage, roast potatoes, carrots OR cheese and
potato pie (see page 279). Banana and tofu cream dessert (see
page 277) with stewed fruit OR baked apple and custard.

## Day 7

### Breakfast
Bran Flakes with 1 dsp topping mix, 200ml milk. Fresh fruit
salad.

### Lunch
Two scrambled eggs on toast OR egg, anchovy and tuna
salad, slice wholemeal bread.
Banana.

### Main Meal
Main meal salad (see page 284) OR pork steak with
cabbage, carrots and 2 boiled potatoes, gravy.
Baked apple filled with raisins, custard.

# Teen Chaos Diet

So you're fed up with being a teenager? Your periods are bad and everyone else can wear the clothes you long for. On top of all the havoc of endless rows with your parents, not having enough money and having to go to school, you're tired all the time, you haven't got the legs you long for and you're made fun of for being fat. Life's tough.

Nobody could understand better than me. I came from a wonderful family, but the total extent of my sex education was for my mother to tell me that school had advised her my periods had started so, 'the things you need are in the airing-cupboard'. That was it! We didn't discuss any feminine issues from that day onwards, and I sort of stumbled my way through boys and period pains and growing breasts and, looking back, I can't say now that I was any the worse for this rather hazy understanding of my hormones.

However, you're growing and changing faster than ever by now, and being healthy is the absolute, complete number-one priority for you. You are lucky enough to be laying down the foundations of your body for the future, and put simply, what you don't do now won't be worth doing in ten years time. Bones for example, are being strengthened now, and your need for calcium is almost as great as it is for a nursing mother. So do take note of my teenage diet and, even if you don't have much influence on the purse-strings in your house, try to eat as much of the right diet as you can.

Being premenstrual at your age is the same as any other age, so do take my tips on water retention and PMS on board. See pages 204 and 229 for tips on what food to eat.

It might be a psychological pressure, but lack of good nutrition is a major cause of low mood, anxiety and sleeplessness. If you suffer from any kind of tearfulness and feelings of hopelessness, I can promise you that a new diet will work wonders without making you fat. See page 187 for the Beat Your Body Chaos diet, which if you are already very lightweight, will have enough calories to help maintain your weight but improve your performance. Remember that your food should be nutrient and energy dense, supplying enough calories for the enormous amount of energy you are using. With the right diet and nutrition you'll feel less tired and have more control especially over your emotions.

I completely understand that you want to stay slim and in tip-top condition. It is my job to be in shape too, but bearing in mind that you can't go through life eating nothing at all, all I want to do is exchange the meals you've been having for meals that fit your lifestyle and special needs a little better. I am not going to introduce calories for the sake of them.

Nutrient tables can be quite offputting. It's a good idea to tell people they need 1000mg of calcium a day and food labels have allowed us at last to know what we're getting, but a kilo of fresh butcher's mince doesn't have a label. The potatoes and sprouts someone's brought you from the allotment don't have labels. So look at the nutrition section in this book and see which foods are the best for calcium and whether you like it or not make sure they're in your diet. You really need calcium – we all do, and plodding on with a junk-food diet in the hope that damage somehow won't happen to you is burying your head in the sand.

## Teenage Diet

### This diet:

- is suitable for teens aged from 14–19
- has approximately 2,000 calories a day
- is energy dense
- is rich in iron
- is rich in protein
- is high in calcium
- means no supplements are necessary

### Shopping list

- fruit spreads, jams and marmalades with no added sugar, do NOT choose those which have artificial sweeteners, ideal brands are St Dalfour, Waitrose own
- eggs
- grapes, apples, bananas, pears, oranges
- plain, live bio yoghurts e.g. Yeo Valley
- mixed whole unsalted nuts e.g. brazils, almonds
- unsweetened muesli e.g. 'Familia' from Health food shops but Sainsbury's unsweetened muesli will do
- Special K
- Cheddar cheese
- all vegetables
- mixed grain or granary loaf
- chicken breasts, mince, steak or casserole beef

### Energy breaks

These would usually be called 'snacks' but this suggests food eaten in a haphazard way – energy breaks should be scheduled and eaten as any main meal.

- hard-boiled egg on 2 slices Ryvita

- slice apricot and almond flapjack (see page 274)
- slice carrot and orange cake (see page 278)
- small pot fruit salad
- banana milkshake
- pot rice pudding (see page 288)
- chunk Cheddar cheese and small bunch grapes or an apple

## Sample Seven-day Menu

Throughout the diet drink only plain or sparkling mineral water, fruit-flavoured mineral water, fruit juice, tea or decaffeinated coffee, milk.

### Day 1

#### Breakfast
150ml glass of fresh orange juice. 40g Special K, 200ml semi-skimmed milk, 1 slice mixed grain toast, olive oil spread, with Marmite or no-added sugar jam or marmalade.

#### Lunch
Ham sandwiches (4 slices of bread) with salad. Slice fruit cake. Apple.

#### Main Meal
Grilled chicken breast in orange marinade (see page 281) (grill another one and put into the fridge as a spare), steamed broccoli, 226g mashed potatoes, 3 tbsp peas. Baked apple with raisins, 1 tbsp ice cream.

### Day 2

#### Breakfast
40g muesli with mixed nuts and seeds, half an apple and half a banana, sliced, 200ml semi-skimmed milk.

**Lunch**
Small cheese and tomato pizza, 12 chips, sliced tomato. Glass of fresh orange or apple juice. Banana.

**Main Meal**
170g portion pasta shapes, topped with sauce of tomatoes, onions and mixed peppers (you can buy a tin), 1 tbsp Parmesan cheese sprinkled over the sauce. Mango and blueberries in plain yoghurt topped with sunflower seeds.

## Day 3

**Breakfast**
30g Special K, 200ml semi-skimmed milk, 2 slices granary toast with Marmite or fruit spread.

**Lunch**
Chicken sandwiches (using grilled chicken breast left over from Day 1), 1 tsp mayonnaise, lettuce, small packet potato crisps. Banana.

**Main Meal**
Portion low-fat shepherd's pie, carrots and peas. Portion ice cream with fresh fruit salad.

## Day 4

**Breakfast**
3 tbsp grapefruit segments, 40g Cornflakes topped with half an apple, sliced, 200ml semi-skimmed milk.

**Lunch**
3 tbsp baked beans with a jacket potato OR on 2 slices wholemeal toast. Glass of fresh orange or apple juice. Gooseberry fool (see page 286).

**Main Meal**
Lamb chop or steak, carrots, mint sauce, 3 boiled potatoes

OR cheese and potato pie (see page 279). Baked apple filled with raisins, 2 tbsp low-fat custard.

## Day 5

### Breakfast
40g muesli with mixed nuts and seeds, apple and half a banana, sliced, 200ml semi-skimmed milk.

### Lunch
Jacket potato with 2 tbsp grated cheese, mixed colourful salad. A pear and some grapes. Small slice fruit cake.

### Main Meal
Pork or beef stir-fry with mixed colourful vegetables e.g. red and yellow peppers, asparagus spears, broccoli florets, etc., soy sauce on 3–4 tbsp boiled rice. Plain yoghurt or fromage frais with 3 tbsp mixed seeds and nuts, 1 tbsp raisins and mango chunks.

## Day 6

### Breakfast
Two boiled or scrambled eggs with 2 slices wholemeal toast. Glass of fresh orange juice.

### Lunch
Small cheese and tomato pizza, jacket potato mixed salad. Glass of fresh orange or apple juice. Apple and banana, small plain fruit and nut chocolate bar.

### Main Meal
Spaghetti bolognese, mixed colourful salad. Banana and low-fat custard.

## Day 7

Day 7 is one day when anything goes!

# Pre-menstrual Body Chaos Diet

I've already talked about the hormone changes that cause PMS, and now's the time to do something about it. These aren't vague, wishy-washy ideas designed to paper over the cracks. I'm not secretly thinking, 'Well, actually, you might just have to put up with it', like the doctor who gave me a knowing look once and shrugged her shoulders. 'To be honest,' she said, 'there's no point in trying to get away without hormones. There's nothing quite like your own oestrogen.'

Well, I'm not so sure. That was the same doctor who offered me anti-depressants for backache, when my anxiety was caused by the fact that I was soon to be making a fitness video and had good reason to be anxious about my own fitness. It's true that nothing is as good as your own oestrogen, but that's like saying an IVF baby isn't like your own. There are a lot of things you can do to alleviate PMS without recourse to drugs or hormones, so read on. As long as you promise yourself to stick to my advice, I promise you'll find relief from all your chaotic symptoms of backache, mood swings and water retention. (I mention sticking with it because so many people don't. They try a week, feel better and go back to their old ways. A month later they say, 'I tried it, but it didn't work!')

## What You Can Do

You should observe the 'three-hour rule' in eating. You need to keep blood-sugar levels steady because it is those fluctuating levels which cause the adrenalin reaction. This makes you nervy, edgy, restless and 'ready for a fight'. Adrenalin is the hormone of storage and it causes glucose to be put down into muscle glycogen. Your body likes to have glucose in very restricted doses, and it looks at the rate of absorption of glucose to see how fast it's coming in. If it's coming in very fast your insulin judges that you must have had a big meal so it puts out a lot of insulin to redress the balance, and your body is constantly trying to second guess how much insulin is made to keep your glucose in the normal range. When you eat unrefined carbohydrates in measured doses your glucose levels are kept finely balanced and don't swing wildly either way, so neither will you have mood swings or extremes in emotion.

If you tend to binge during low moments or simply out of boredom you might also find that you get more infections than other people. The reasons for this are quite complicated, but basically it's down to insulin release again. As you know, insulin is released in large amounts when you've just had a massive rush of sugar, either from eating, say, chocolates or from a big dose of unrefined carbohydrate like pasta. Your body releases two hormones, adrenalin and cortisol. Cortisol is one of the hormones that suppresses your immune system. So you're eating unrefined carbohydrates and crave more, this makes you fat, knocks your immune system on the head and you keep getting a massive adrenalin rush. Because you've had this massive release of glucose you also release a bit of endorphin which is a neurotransmitter in the brain, a bit like heroin in that it is a painkiller and makes you feel good. So you get addicted and the whole ghastly cycle starts all over again.

I must emphasize that you aren't going to start this diet on Day 1 and miraculously feel fantastic by Day 3. This diet takes time, but it is successful. So give it two complete months at first, starting the diet at the beginning of the fortnight following ovulation, which is usually about Day 14 in your cycle. This is when the hormone progesterone starts to increase its levels. Follow the diet for four weeks to start with, even when you feel fine, and this way you will build yourself up nutritionally for your next bout of PMS.

Remember that these meals are low glycaemic index because you must keep your blood-sugar levels steady. For the two weeks following your period you can eat 'normally' if you choose, although if your symptoms are bad you might want to stick to the principles for good.

## The Basics

- There is an altered glucose tolerance in the few days leading up to your period, and you will be more sensitive to different levels of blood sugar. This can result in outpourings of adrenalin and possible panic attacks, aggression and irritability, leading to tears. So the idea is to keep blood-sugar levels even and to avoid sudden swings in sugar.

- You should observe the three-hour starch diet outlined in the Good Mood Diet (see page 218).

- Make sure that your carbohydrates are mainly of the low glycaemic index type (see page 304).

- Eat within an hour of waking, and an hour before going to bed.

- Your main foods:

| Best | OK | Eat Sparingly |
| --- | --- | --- |
| oats | natural yoghurt | parsnips |
| oranges | potatoes | pineapple |
| pasta | banana | melon |
| pulses | fresh apricots | raisins |

| Best | OK | Eat Sparingly |
|------|-----|---------------|
| apples | sultanas | beetroot |
| cherries | carrots | potatoes |
| grapefruit | baked beans | all biscuits |
| pears | kidney beans | most soups |
| lentil soup (see page 282) | grapes | frozen broad beans |

- Other foods which will help:
  Celery, parsley, asparagus are naturally diuretic and help rid you of retained water.
  Figs, leafy green vegetables, nuts, pulses are magnesium-rich foods. The body tends to be low in magnesium in PMS sufferers.
  Milk, bananas, turkey, cottage cheese are calming foods (see anti-stress diet, page 218).

This is not a weight-loss diet. If you also want to reduce weight, observe the same meals and three-hour starch rules, but reduce portion sizes by a third.

| MONDAY | WEEK ONE | WEEK TWO |
|--------|----------|----------|
| **Breakfast** | 30g unsweetened muesli. 150 ml skimmed milk. One sliced apple. | 150ml fresh orange juice. Two slices granary toast, spread. Boiled egg. |
| **Mid-morning** | Satsuma, banana. | Twelve grapes, pear. |
| **Lunch** | Lentil soup (see page 282) with wholemeal roll. Apple. | Tuna and pasta salad with mixed peppers, cucumber dice. Natural yoghurt with blackberries. |
| **Three-hour Break** | Slice home-made date and walnut cake (see page 279). | Two oat biscuits, glass skimmed milk. |

| | | |
|---|---|---|
| **Main Meal** | Shepherd's pie (without the potato), sprouts, peas, broccoli.<br>Baked apple with 1 tsp raisins. | Home-made meatballs in tomato sauce (see page 284), broccoli, 84g pasta shapes. Baked apple with 1tbsp raisins. |
| **Bedtime Snack** | Small bowl (30g) porridge made with water and 2 dsp milk or half-fat, evaporated milk . | 56g unsweetened popcorn. |

| **TUESDAY** | **WEEK ONE** | **WEEK TWO** |
|---|---|---|
| **Breakfast** | 30g unsweetened muesli, 150ml skimmed milk. One banana. | Citrus salad. 30g Special K, 150ml skimmed milk. One banana. |
| **Mid-morning** | Apricot and almond flapjack (see page 274). | One slice granary toast, Marmite. |
| **Lunch** | Lentil or tomato soup, small granary roll. Natural fromage frais with fruit compote. | Chicken and avocado salad with Basmati rice and curried mayonnaise. Banana, apple and grape salad. |
| **Three-hour Break** | 150ml banana milk shake. | Small pot (150 ml) home-made rice pudding (see page 288). |
| **Main Meal** | 170g stir-fried chicken, mixed cooked salad (see page 285). Sweet Marscapone mousse (see page 294). | Pasta with green vegetable sauce (see page 286). Sweet Marscapone mousse (see page 289). |
| **Bedtime Snack** | Small slice chocolate cake. Apple. | Small slice chocolate cake. Apple. |

| WEDNESDAY | WEEK ONE | WEEK TWO |
| --- | --- | --- |
| **Breakfast** | Two scrambled eggs on one slice granary toast. One banana. | 2 tbsp grapefruit segments. Two slices wholemeal toast, 2 tsp no-added sugar spread. |
| **Mid-morning** | Fruit bread slice, toasted. | Natural yoghurt with 3 chopped apricots, 1 tsp raisins, tsp chopped mixed nuts. |
| **Lunch** | 250ml tomato soup with granary roll. Sliced apple in natural yoghurt. | 250ml lentil soup (see page 282) with granary roll. Home-made blackcurrant fromage frais. |
| **Three-hour Break** | 150ml banana milk shake. | 150ml banana milk shake. |
| **Main Meal** | Two-egg Spanish omelette (see page 287) with salad, 2 tbsp sweetcorn. Stewed apples with fromage frais. | Seafood risotto with peas. Stewed apples with fromage frais. |
| **Bedtime Snack** | Small bowl (30g) porridge made with water and 2 dsp milk or half-fat evaporated milk added. | Small pot rice pudding (see page 288) |

| THURSDAY | WEEK ONE | WEEK TWO |
| --- | --- | --- |
| **Breakfast** | 30g unsweetened muesli, 150ml skimmed milk. One banana | Citrus salad. 30g Special K, 150ml skimmed milk. One banana. |
| **Mid-morning** | Bowl fresh fruit salad. | Bowl fresh fruit salad. |
| **Lunch** | Cold chicken with Basmati rice, 2 tsp mayonnaise. Apple. | 2 tbsp tuna in brine with 2 tbsp peas, 1 tbsp mayonnaise, few chopped peppers. Apple. |

| **Three-hour Break** | Banana milk shake. | Small slice banana cake (see page 276). |
| **Main Meal** | 170g stir-fried chicken, 85g pasta shapes, mixed cooked salad (see page 290). Sweet Marscapone mousse (see page 289). | Pasta with green vegetable sauce (see page 286). Sweet Marscapone mousse (see page 289). |
| **Bedtime Snack** | Small bowl (30g) porridge made with water and 2 dsp milk or half-fat evaporated milk added. | 30g All Bran, 150ml skimmed milk. Half apple, sliced. |

| **FRIDAY** | **WEEK ONE** | **WEEK TWO** |
| --- | --- | --- |
| **Breakfast** | 30g All Bran topped with half banana, sliced, 200ml skimmed milk | 40g porridge topped with 1 tbsp raisins, little milk, 2 tbsp grapefruit segments. |
| **Mid-morning** | Slice banana cake (see page 276). | One slice granary toast, Marmite. |
| **Lunch** | Fruit muffin or bap filled with either sliced banana and topped with 1 tsp crème fraiche OR plain muffin split and toasted, with 2 tbsp baked beans. | 113g cold chicken on 3 tbsp cold Basmati rice, dressed with 1 tsp mayonnaise and 6 sliced grapes. Apple. |
| **Three-hour Break** | 150ml banana milk shake. | 150ml home-made rice pudding (see page 288). |
| **Main Meal** | 170g cod or haddock fillet, steamed carrots, peas, broccoli. Portion hot rice pudding topped with stewed apple. | 170g salmon fillet, poached, steamed vegetables as last week. Fresh fruit salad without pineapple or melon. |

| SATURDAY | WEEK ONE | WEEK TWO |
|---|---|---|
| **Bedtime Snack** | 30g All Bran topped with half apple sliced, orange segments, 150ml skimmed milk | Small portion banana topped with rice pudding (see page 288). |
| **Breakfast** | 30g unsweetened muesli, 150ml skimmed milk. One banana. | Citrus salad. 30g Special K, 150ml skimmed milk. |
| **Mid-morning** | Apricot and almond flapjack (see page 274). | One slice granary toast, Marmite. |
| **Lunch** | 170g jacket potato with 2 tbsp baked beans, salad. Banana and 2 tbsp custard made without sugar, use artificial sweetener. | Tuna sandwich made with 2 slices granary bread, 1 tsp mayonnaise, plenty of watercress. Natural yoghurt with compote topping. |
| **Three-hour Break** | 150ml banana milk shake. | 150 ml rice pudding (see page 288). |
| **Main Meal** | Chicken vindaloo with Basmati rice mixed colourful salad. Sweet Marscapone mousse (see page 289) | Chilli con carne with Basmati rice mixed colourful salad. Sweet Marscapone mousse (see page 289). |
| **Bedtime Snack** | 200ml mug of warm skimmed milk with 1 tsp sugar OR milky decaffeinated coffee. Apple. | One Shredded Wheat, no sugar, 150ml skimmed milk, half apple sliced. |

| SUNDAY | WEEK 1 | WEEK 2 |
|---|---|---|
| **Breakfast** | One poached egg, 1 rasher bacon. Glass fresh orange juice. One slice toast and spread. | 30g Sustain, 1 boiled egg. Glass fresh orange juice. One slice toast and spread. |

| | | |
|---|---|---|
| **Mid-morning** | One banana. | Apricot and almond flapjack (see page 274). |
| **Lunch** | (Same lunch both weeks)<br>Sunday lunch of 113g roast beef or chicken, 2 tbsp peas, carrots, broccoli, 1 dsp stuffing, 2 tbsp gravy, broccoli. Stewed mixed fruit with custard or a little half-fat cream. | |
| **Three-hour Break** | 30g mixed fruit and nuts (not salted). | 150 ml rice pudding (see page 288). |
| **Light Meal** | Salad sandwich. Slice chocolate cake. Bowl fresh fruit salad. | Ham salad. Slice home-made fruit cake. Fresh fruit salad. |
| **Bedtime Snack** | 200ml mug of warm skimmed milk OR Shredded Wheat, no sugar. 150ml milk, 1 tsp sugar OR milky decaffeinated coffee. One apple. | 2 Ryvitas with honey. 200ml warm skimmed milk. Half apple sliced. |

## Pre-menstrual Comfort Eating and Bingeing Chaos

These are problems which need a strategy for coping, 'tricks of the trade' and small changes in your routine, rather than just a diet. Have a think about these ideas:

– Get out of the house, find something to do. If you can't take up another activity, ask yourself these questions:

- When you last had a lot to eat, did you enjoy it?
- If you managed to resist food now, how would you feel, good or bad?
- You call it 'comfort eating' but does it comfort you?

– Eat later. This is the best solution if you really can't help yourself. You have two options:

- Save your entire evening meal until about 9 p.m.
- Eat half now, and save the other half until 9–10 p.m.

– Get a lightbox or have more walks. The cure for many winter carbohydrate cravings is to get a lightbox. I have one, and you can find companies which supply them in the 'Lighting' section of *Yellow Pages*. Expect to pay between £70 and £150 at the time of writing, although trends in what is called 'Full Spectrum Lighting' are growing all the time, and I daresay prices will come down. In the dark winter mornings you simply put it in front of you for about half an hour to an hour, then you can carry on as normal with your day. If you prefer, take every opportunity to walk in daylight, and it doesn't have to be sunny. If you work in artificial light, get out at lunchtime and make sure you spend at least half an hour outdoors. Put your desk by a window. Don't stay in bed until lunchtime at weekends. Get as much daylight as you can and I promise you'll soon find the cravings diminish, and you'll begin to lose weight into the bargain.

– Go with the flow. The hormones around the time of your period are encouraging a nest-building phase, so if you want to eat, don't fight it. Trying not to eat means it becomes all the more tempting. Plan an extra 500 calories in substantial meals (not just bars of chocolate or junk foods) and stay on this plan for your five worst days. You will have eaten just 2,500 extra calories, a thousand less than half a kilo of fat! Going to tell me that you stepped on the scales and you'd gained 2.25kg? It's not fat I promise, it's water. If you don't believe me, to gain an extra 2.25kg of fat you'd have had to have eaten your normal 2,000 calories every day for five days PLUS another 17,500 calories, a grand total of 27,500 calories. However much you think you can eat for England, I think even this would be a bit of a challenge!

– Change your territory, I've said this before but it really is important. This includes the people you associate with.

Fine, you won't want to ditch all your best friends simply because you can't resist food, but ask yourself if they're really helping? Some friends are habits. Some friends belong to another time, and they might be encouraging you along the wrong path. 'You look fine as you are!' is one unhelpful phrase, along with, 'Come on, you've got to die of something!' I've got a few more of these in the Mental Chaos section, but do take time to think through your routine. Places also fall into this category and times of eating. I can't be specific because I don't know you, but it's not difficult to break down your territorial connections. Here are some other ideas:

- Go to work by another route.
- Shop after you've eaten, not when you're hungry.
- If you cave in, forgive yourself immediately – don't make one lapse the reason you go on and eat the fridge bare!

## Pregnancy Chaos Diet

Pregnancy can be a chaotic time for your hormones, but after the first few weeks most women settle down to some of the most glowing months they've ever experienced! The advice I can give you for this stage in your life is brief: pregnancy lasts just nine months, and compared with the years of teenage and menopausal chaos, you've got it made. As any mother will tell you, it isn't so much the pregnancy that brings chaos, but the months afterwards. Many women find that their pre-pregnancy weight and figure vanishes never to be seen again, but it needn't be like that. I recently wrote a diet leaflet after a story of a shapely young girl who'd gone completely to pot after her baby was born, and

I have never had such an overwhelming response. It seems that just like I said in the introduction, you are your own best friend. The longest relationship you will have with anybody is with yourself, and looking in the mirror and not recognizing the person who looks back at you is frightening. Whenever I see a carefree, laughing young girl now, stuffing herself with chips without a care in the world, I fast-forward in my mind to the pleading letters of these young mothers and I think, 'Watch out – don't take yourself for granted!'

But now you are pregnant and you need to take care of not just yourself, but the little one growing inside you.

## Nutritional Facts

### Weeks 13–26

From week 13, the foetus grows dramatically. By week 26 the baby will weigh between half to one kilo and measure about 28–36 cm. This time of vital growth and development means that your requirement of calories, minerals, vitamins and protein increases significantly.

### Protein

From week 13, more protein is needed to support the rapid growth of the baby, to form the placenta and increase your blood volume. Make sure that you eat enough carbo-hydrate, because without it your body will burn protein for energy, leaving your stores low. I suggest you eat about 75–100g protein a day.

### Calcium

You need more calcium during pregnancy as it is responsible for building bone and regulating muscle and nerve function. You need about 1000mg calcium a day, but if you don't drink milk you can still get enough calcium from salmon, sardines or leafy green vegetables.

## Iron

Iron is important during pregnancy because if the baby doesn't have enough, it will take its stores from you, leaving you even more tired than you were before. It is not always beneficial to take supplements because they can cause constipation, and doctors these days are cautious about prescribing them. There's no need for supplements if you eat enough meat, spinach, raisins and dried apricots.

## Calorie needs and weight gain in pregnancy

What you eat in pregnancy should add up to a healthy weight gain:

- First three months – your weight should hardly change.
- Last six months – you need an extra 300 calories a day.
- If you were a normal weight when you got pregnant you should gain about 9–11kg.
- If you were overweight when you got pregnant you should gain 7–9kg.
- If you were underweight when you got pregnant you should gain 12–18kg.
- If you are having twins aim to gain around 16–21kg.

## Foods to avoid

To be on the safe side you should avoid the following while you're pregnant:

- soft cheese like Brie, Camembert, feta
- caffeine
- seafood
- alcohol
- nuts are an issue, but the General Medical Council suggest that you should only avoid them if a close relative has suffered from a peanut allergy, otherwise, you are safe to consume normal portions of nuts

## Sample Seven-day Menu

### Day 1

**Breakfast**
One egg, scrambled on 1 slice toast. Glass of fresh orange juice.

**Mid-morning**
Hot chocolate, apple.

**Lunch**
Houmous in pitta bread with shredded carrot, lettuce, tomato. Fresh fruit salad.

**Mid-afternoon**
25g roasted almonds, glass apple juice.

**Main Meal**
Cod or plaice on spinach, cauliflower, 2 boiled potatoes. Meringue with fresh fruit and topped with plain live yoghurt.

### Day 2

**Breakfast**
40g porridge, skimmed milk, 1 tsp sugar, 2 slices whole-wheat toast, 2 tsp marmalade, a little olive oil spread. Glass of fresh orange juice.

**Mid-morning**
Salad sandwich, apple.

**Lunch**
Two-egg herb omelette, 2 tbsp baked beans. Fromage frais with chopped apple or sliced strawberries.

**Mid-afternoon**
Two Ryvitas topped with low-fat cottage cheese.

**Main Meal**
Cauliflower cheese, jacket potato, 2 sliced tomatoes. Meringue with fresh fruit and topped with plain live yoghurt.

## Day 3

**Breakfast**
56g tofu blended with half a banana topped with tin strawberries or 8 fresh strawberries, 1 bran muffin, toasted. Glass of fresh orange juice.

**Mid-morning**
Sesame-seed roll spread with peanut butter or Marmite.

**Lunch**
Wholewheat pitta filled with mixed beans and tomatoes, sliced, little grated Cheddar cheese. Apple.

**Mid-afternoon**
Two oatcakes with sugar-free spread. Glass of skimmed milk.

**Main Meal**
Stir-fried vegetable curry (see page 288) with brown rice. Fresh fruit salad.

## Day 4

**Breakfast**
30g Bran Flakes, 150ml skimmed milk, half a banana and an apple, sliced.

**Mid-morning**
Two carrots cut into sticks, 50g cottage cheese.

**Lunch**
Chicken or tuna sandwich with shredded lettuce and carrot, sliced tomato. An orange.

### Mid-afternoon
25g roasted almonds, glass of apple juice.

### Main Meal
Cod or plaice on spinach, cauliflower, 2 boiled potatoes. Meringue with fresh fruit and topped with plain live yoghurt.

## Day 5

### Breakfast
Two boiled eggs, 2 rashers bacon, grilled tomato, 2 slices wholewheat toast, olive oil spread. Glass of fresh orange juice.

### Mid-morning
Cappuccino or latte, slice apricot and almond flapjack (see page 274).

### Lunch
Mixed salad with mackerel or tuna. An apple.

### Mid-afternoon
Twenty twiglets, glass banana shake made with soya milk.

### Main Meal
Roast chicken, dry-roast potatoes, broccoli, cauliflower, carrots. Meringue topped with 1 scoop ice cream.

## Day 6

### Breakfast
40g oat-based muesli, skimmed milk. 1 bran muffin with olive oil spread.

### Mid-morning
Hot chocolate, apple.

### Lunch
Ham salad sandwich or egg mayonnaise sandwich on

granary bread with shredded lettuce. Fruit yoghurt (see page 280).

### Mid-afternoon
Slice carrot and orange cake (see page 278). Milky coffee or glass skimmed milk blended with strawberries.

### Main Meal
Wholewheat spaghetti bolognese made at home with tomatoes, peppers and onions and very low-fat minced beef, mixed side salad. Stewed apple or rhubarb with custard.

## Day 7

### Breakfast
40g Sustain, skimmed milk, 1 boiled egg, slice granary toast. Glass of fresh orange juice.

### Mid-morning
Banana and sliced grapes, mixed.

### Lunch
Roast beef, gravy, Yorkshire pudding, three vegetables OR vegetarian lasagne with side serving of mixed, stir-fried vegetables. Slice of apple pie or crumble, custard or cream.

### Mid-afternoon
Slice apricot and almond flapjack (see page 274), apple.

### Light meal
Half ciabatta topped with tomatoes and peppers, grilled, sprinkled with Parmesan cheese. Fresh fruit salad.

## Mid-life Chaos Diet

'Retired from my job – not from life!'

It's the familiar cry of many middle-aged women, 'I've just got my life together and my body is falling apart!' You've spent your youth simultaneously drinking yourself under the table, frying yourself to a crisp in the midday sun, smoking up a storm and eating rubbish, and you still had time to put in a day's work. Life was something to get through, to enjoy or to endure, but what you certainly never stopped to think about was the future. Then suddenly it all falls into place. Your finances are sorted, the children leave home and you reach the top of your career. You have the time and the money to go out and enjoy yourself but there's that twinge in the back and those baggy eyes. Your mind's that of a teenager but your body's that of a pensioner. Short of handing over a substantial cheque to a willing plastic surgeon, you're stuck with it. Over the hill, washed-up and past it.

Middle age conjures up a grey image. I even read a fashion article the other day which advised women in their forties to 'be careful to hide those iffy bits in the middle'. Well, speak for yourself, because when it comes to 'iffy bits' I've seen just as many coming out of our local comprehensive school gates as I have in a roomful of fifty-somethings. Looking good doesn't belong to the young and the goalposts have moved.

On the plus side, having a houseful of chattering teenagers to stop you feeling redundant means the sort of social life where you might feel pleasantly competitive with the other parents. But we're not all parents, and whether or not you're happily child-free or gratefully clearing out the empty nest, you still want to be attractive and enjoy yourself in whatever way does it for you. After all, these days if you're forty you could easily be looking at another forty years. Life's too short they say, but couldn't it also be a bit too long? How are you going to fill all those years? What challenges have you ahead, and how are you going to cope with them?

## In Good Working Order

If you were to set off on an extended world trip by caravan, your first priority would be to make sure your vehicle was in tip-top condition, and the same applies to the kind of nick you keep yourself in. Your metabolism has been changing for at least fifteen years and most letters I get from women over the age of fifty express despair about their weight and their waistline. Unless you are on HRT, your oestrogen will have dwindled considerably by now, and that leads to weight redistribution. You might not weigh more, but your figure might have gone distinctly apple-shaped. Most women complain about menopausal weight gain, but believe me, I have explored this topic as much as it's possible for a human being to do, and I have come to the conclusion that while anecdotal evidence suggests there is weight gain on hormone replacement, there is still no firm evidence for it and I don't believe that the hormones are responsible.

Tackling mid-life chaos means taking several steps:

1. Get your diet right. Absolutely NO excess calories of any kind, fatty acids from seeds and nuts, carbohydrates reduced by 10 per cent.

2. Exercise as much as possible. Don't just say you'll do it, make a PLAN, and commit to it.

3. Keep yourself in good order. That means never having a day with unwashed hair or sloppy clothes. You'll only drag yourself down mentally.

4. Stop smoking.


## Coping With Hot Flushes

Hot flushes can drag you down no end. You can deal with them quite easily with a few strategies for making them no more or less than a vague nuisance. Your plan of action for bad hot-flush days is:

1. Have a bath or shower, wash your hair and apply a little make-up. If you have no time, wash your hair only. Time spent on getting yourself in reasonable order is never wasted because it is psychologically necessary to feel attractive and in control of your looks.

2. Keep the house at a temperature of 19 C. If it is winter, wear light layers of clothes and cardigan or jacket which can be taken off without disturbing your hair.

3. If it is impossible to keep a cool house because other family members object, explain the situation and keep one room for yourself which is either cold or very cool. This can become your retreat.

4. Get your own bed, or buy two single duvets. You must accept that this is a difficult time but no worse than having a new baby in the house, and sharing a bed for the sake of it when you're both being disturbed isn't going to help. If you have to share, don't share bedclothes.

5. Don't drink alcohol. You'll only get hot hands and feet which will make matters a lot worse.

6. Keep a glass of iced water or juice handy. When a flush comes, it will be easier to have a sip of an iced drink than stand out in the snow!

7. Keep a proper orthopaedic ice-pack handy. They are kept in the freezer, are soft, and they keep cold for ages, so put it by your chair and slip it inside your blouse when you feel a flush starting. It is incredibly soothing. You can buy these packs at chiropractic clinics.

8. Eat a good diet which includes soya protein, linseeds, vitamin E and evening primrose oil – these have plant oestrogens which, although in tiny amounts, are known to relieve the severest symptoms of flushes and night sweats. The herbal remedy red clover is also thought to be beneficial.

9. See your doctor to discuss HRT if symptoms are too bad to handle.

10. Don't panic. Hot flushes don't go on all the time and you'll get a certain amount of time off. If you panic and think that this is the end of the world as you know it, your flushes will get worse. There are currently more women aged fifty than the entire 16–19 age group put together, so thousands of women somewhere are having hot flushes at the same time as you.

## Diet for Years Leading up to the Menopause

### Energy breaks – choose no more than two a day

- two oatcakes with no-sugar spread
- banana
- small date slice
- slice apricot and almond flapjack (see page 274)

- carrot and celery sticks with 1 tbsp houmous
- two Ryvitas with cottage cheese or sugar-free spread
- two pieces of any fruit
- two Ryvitas with peanut butter

## Sample Seven-day Menu

Every day take 1 vitamin E tablet, 1 evening primrose capsule, 3 red clover tablets, 1 cod liver oil capsule.

### Day 1

**Breakfast**
30g Cornflakes, 1 tsp wheatgerm, tsp linseeds, half an apple, sliced, 150ml skimmed milk (soya milk if you are near the menopause). Herbal tea or decaffeinated coffee.

**Lunch**
Sardines on 1 slice toast OR 1 tbsp tuna in oil with 85g (cooked weight) pasta shapes, mixed peppers. Small pot soya yoghurt topped with a little stewed apple.

**Main Meal**
Stir-fried mixed vegetables, including broccoli, 170g chicken or pork or quorn. Bio yoghurt with tsp linseeds, tsp raisins.

### Day 2

**Breakfast**
2 tbsp grapefruit segments, 2 slices mixed grain bread, olive oil spread, Marmite or sugar-free spread.

**Lunch**
Potato, salad of chopped celery, pine nuts, lettuce with olive oil and lemon juice dressing. Banana and apple slices mixed.

**Main Meal**
Tofu or chicken kebabs with peppers, mushrooms, broccoli and courgettes. 2 tbsp rice pudding (see page 288) with tsp linseeds.

## Day 3

**Breakfast**
Glass of fresh orange juice. 30g muesli, 150ml skimmed milk, topped with grapes.

**Lunch**
Two scrambled eggs on 1 slice wholemeal toast, apple OR main meal salad (see page 284).

**Main Meal**
Warm chicken or beef salad (see page 292) on bed of salad leaves, with stir-fried red and yellow peppers. Portion ice cream.

## Day 4

**Breakfast**
Glass of fresh orange juice. One boiled egg with 2 slices mixed grain bread.

**Lunch**
113g tuna in oil, topping a mixed salad with chicory leaves, asparagus spears, slices of orange (to taste) and shredded lettuce. A slice of sundried tomato or olive bread OR 170g jacket potato. Pot soya yoghurt with sliced apple.

**Main Meal**
Poached salmon fillet (make one spare) with 3 tbsp peas, sweetcorn (make extra spare), broccoli and carrots, 2 boiled new potatoes. Fresh fruit salad with 1 scoop ice cream.

## Day 5

### Breakfast
Muesli with linseeds, few whole hazelnuts, 150ml skimmed milk.

### Lunch
Salad of cold peas and sweetcorn on salad greens topped with flaked cold salmon (from last night) oil and vinegar dressing. Pear and few grapes.

### Main Meal
Two-egg cheese omelette or Spanish omelette (see page 287) with broccoli. Banana and tofu cream dessert (see page 277).

## Day 6

### Breakfast
Grapefruit segments. Bacon sandwich OR Cornflakes and 150ml skimmed or soya milk.

### Lunch
Tuna fish sandwich on granary with salad and 1 tsp oil and lemon dressing. Banana milk shake.

### Main Meal
Chilli con carne with Basmati rice OR vegetable chilli (see page 291) with a mixed colourful salad. Meringue filled with strawberries and blueberries.

## Day 7

This is a day to eat whatever takes your fancy but you must have your daily supplements.

# Weight-Gain Diet

Weight gain isn't talked about as much as weight loss, but whenever I write about it I get a bigger mailbag than I ever get about weight loss. People who are too thin feel isolated and picked on. They are targets of inappropriate remarks and thoughtless jibes. People will invade the psychological space of the thin person in a way they'd never dare to do if the person concerned was fat. Magazines declare open season on actresses and models who are thin, and the depths of rudeness some journalists think they can sink to takes my breath away. In a nutshell, I don't think someone's dress size or weight is anybody else's business.

Weight gain needs to be done with care if you are to avoid gaining 'fat weight' which can collect anywhere on your body and you have no control over it – for example on your back, face or ankles! The idea is to weight-train your muscles, and eat a diet which has enough nutrient- and energy-dense components to help them develop.

NB – If you try to eat this diet and not exercise, you will gain fat and not improve your shape.

This diet example is for one day, and supplies approximately 2,500 calories. You must drink 2.25 litres of water (minimum) every day.

### Breakfast
Porridge made with water, 1 tsp golden syrup or sugar. One slice wholemeal toast with honey, no butter or spread. One banana.

### Mid-morning
One banana, 1 apple. One slice toast, no butter. Glass of fresh orange juice.

### Lunch
Jacket potato. Grilled or cold chicken breast and salad OR 170g tuna in brine, mixed salad and hard-boiled egg. Jelly with plain bio yoghurt and fruit.

### Mid-afternoon
One slice wholemeal toast, Marmite, jacket potato, 56g low-fat cottage cheese. Banana. Glass of fresh orange juice.

### Evening Meal
226g boiled pasta or rice and curried vegetables with chicken or tomato sauce OR 226g potatoes, grilled chicken or lamb, vegetables. Fruit salad with 2 scoops of ice cream.

### Mid-evening
Glass of skimmed milk, 2 slices toast, Marmite. One apple.

# Chapter Ten

# Exercise: I want to look Gorgeous

We were built to last – but not indefinitely. Primitive man was made for survival, with the ability to walk for an entire day to find food and water. To imagine that an endurance trek of fifty miles is somehow beyond you physically is to misunderstand the function of your body. The only difference between then and now is that we live longer than we were meant to live, and so we experience more damage, wear and tear and mobility problems than our ancestors did.

Consider how we treat these joints and powerful muscles which should enable us to climb mountains and cross rivers: we put them in armchairs. We limit our impressive range of joint mobility to a few everyday actions like craning round to reverse the car or bending to feed the cat. If you are suffering from body chaos of the painful kind, could it be that it's time to loosen up a little?

But this isn't a lecture on your shortcomings. Whatever limitations we've placed on our bodies, we've managed to increase our lifespan. If ancient man had lived as long he would have lived a life of brittle bones and osteoarthritis; without much starch in his diet, he would also have suffered the damaging effects of ketosis on his kidneys. By contrast, you have a brilliant opportunity to make the most of your body through easy exercise, which doesn't even need a favourable weather forecast.

When you look back to the glamorous fashions of the thirties and fifties, or the super-slim figures of the sixties, don't you ever wonder how all those women managed it with only the municipal swimming pool, ballet classes and the odd game of tennis to help them? Keep fit classes certainly existed for those with the leisure time and the cash, but most women stayed slim and glamorous through a much more active daily life, and the duty to themselves to look as good as possible. The words 'I'm slimming' were on everybody's lips without it suddenly becoming an eating disorder, and doing your 'daily dozen' – a term used to describe a set of stretching and mobility exercises was how most women looked after their curves. So now that almost anybody can afford to join a gym, and spend as often as they like with children in tow, how come the nation is fatter, flabbier and weaker?

The modern craze for exercise has made it seem more like a dose of medicine than an enjoyable pastime. You are told to exercise for your heart, lungs, fat stores or muscle flexibility, but exercise as a pleasant way to spend your leisure is relegated to a secondary benefit. Yet the quality of your life is deeply influenced by your capacity to perform basic activities without pain or strain. You might think that you don't wish to prune a high branch or climb over a gate but that's because you take these capabilities for granted. Being physically able is one of the greatest freedoms you can have because freedom means choice. A poor capacity for physical enjoyment closes the door on many enjoyable pursuits, and this sets up a vicious circle of inactivity and worse, deterioration. On the other hand, if you make a real effort to get fitter, things get better. I am not against the benefits of gym-based exercise such as weight training and exercise bikes, and if you live in a built-up area or need to exercise at times when lack of daylight or poor weather conditions make it unpleasant to exercise outdoors, indoor exercise is sensible and certainly better than not doing it at all. Going to a gym has the compensations of meeting people and getting the kind of motivation you can only get from a class of like-minded people – and I'm all for that. But don't rely on a gym session to solve all your weight and figure problems. Five hours a week might sound impressive, but if you are trying to make up for an entire week of sitting on your bottom and eating and drinking badly, you'll be disappointed. Even if you really go for it and kill yourself on the rowing machine or treadmill, you could burn 10–12 calories a minute for those five hours, a reasonable 3,000–3,600 calories which is exactly half a kilo of fat. If you did five hours of aerobics you would burn just 1,800 calories in the whole week, easily replaced by just two substantial Indian takeaways. I don't know about you, but I'd rather not spend half an hour eating an Indian meal if it takes two and a half hours of aerobics to make up for it. But of course exercise is about more than the number of calories you use. If you enjoy it, carry on doing it.

If you don't have the physical capability to join others or do whatever takes your whim, your life will be limited, and this is a particularly sore point when you are young. One somehow expects or is not surprised if a middle-aged or old woman can't climb stairs or take to the dance floor but when you are a teenager it automatically draws attention to you. Being out of step makes you feel inadequate, and I have read thousands of letters from anguished young women who feel this isolation acutely. They will say that it is their weight or the size of a certain part of their body which gives rise to their feelings, but it is more likely to be the alienation from their group. So does exercise have to be taken like a dose of protective medicine, or accepted as you might the job of washing your hair?

All types of activity are exercise:

- Exercise deliberately chosen for pleasure – football, tennis, swimming.
- Exercise for health – deep breathing, yoga.

- The inescapable part of living exercise – mowing the lawn, carrying shopping, walking the dog.
- Exercising for a living – the postman, horse-rider, gardener.

Small children are spontaneously active. Play and exploration are the mainstay of a child's life, but when you reach your teens you have better things to do with your time, and throwing yourself around a hockey pitch plays havoc with your hair! Recent reports that teenage girls spent less time in sporting activities were met by guffaws from most of us – of course they do! I never enjoyed being active once I'd reached my teens, mostly because of self-consciousness about my body, plus you're never going to impress a boy when you're dressed in hockey socks and an aertex blouse. Mind you, in my school days exercise was seen as the cure for everything, and woe betide you if you appeared in your Latin class doubled up with a period pain because you'd be shunted off to join the nearest netball session. Sitting here now I think it was sound advice, the purpose of which was to mask agony with a burst of painkilling endorphins. It was a ploy which worked and developed in us a strong streak of stoicism! But good looks just don't get ordered up on the telephone. You can spend as many hours as you like in the bathroom using the costly miracle hair thickener you just bought, but it won't make an atom of difference if your hair's in rotten condition because you eat like a child. You can spend all your birthday money on those trousers you were mad for, but if your thighs are lumpy because you never get out of your armchair, you might as well tear up your money. The fact is, you can't buy a good body, nails or hair. You have to grow them.

## Never Too Late

It is never too late to start an exercise programme. Looking good and being fit is not the exclusive domain of the young, and middle-age spread or weight gain after a baby are not inevitable. Many women find their bodies refine as they get older, losing so-called 'puppy-fat'. The inevitable stresses and strains that come with this upward shift can mean that for many women, looks, weight and figure improve rather than diminish.

What is inescapable though, is the consistency of any routine you get yourself into. You can't put improvements into some kind of bank, making the most, as it were, of the times when you feel like exercising so you can have a few weeks off. If you embark on a fitness regime for a special event like a holiday, and then you go back to your old ways afterwards, your old shape will come back. Having said that, the effort it takes to stay in shape is nowhere near as great as it is to get there in the first place. As an analogy, I am reminded of the days when I used to go to a local gym where there were many young male bodybuilders. Night after night they would turn up and go through a rigorous, gut-busting routine, but three times a week Keith came in. Keith was a middle-aged businessman, and although he wasn't a fitness professional his physique meant a lot to him, he'd trained for twenty years and was in fantastic, jaw-dropping shape. We all watched as he ambled in, warmed up, then started on the heaviest weights in the gym. He did a few lifts, took a breather, did a few more in different positions, then ambled off again. His entire routine took fifteen minutes and the place came to a halt. He was a marvellous example of only needing a short, sharp routine to maintain the changes rather than improve on them, and the secret of his success was the regularity with which he did this. And like Keith, regularity and consistency are the keys to your success.

So don't be slack for two weeks and then try to make up for it with a two-hour run or back-to-back aerobics classes. Apart from the fact that this is the quickest way to get injuries, your body works on a steady, rhythmic basis.

Don't just dream it – do it!

## Finding Time

The biggest hurdle for most people is finding the time for an exercise programme, but if you try to find time you'll never do it. The basic rule of course is that anything is better than nothing, but then that can be used as an excuse for doing as little as possible. You must push yourself. People will often say to me, 'Can you give me an exercise plan which gets me in shape quickly?' Yes, I can give them a quick exercise plan, but it won't have the same effect as one which devotes a little more time to it. On the other hand, pounding away in a gym for two hours at a time does no more for you, and can even do harm. The general rule is to exercise four, concentrated sessions, of 40–50 minutes each week, and in between times be very active in a general way, such as walking.

Here are my tips for managing your time more effectively:

1. Be honest – how bad is your body chaos? How much do you hate those bits of yourself which you're ashamed of? Being successful depends largely on how important it is to you.

2. You can't squeeze more time out of your schedule, so instead of making time, you must stop doing something else and start doing this.

3. Be realistic about the television programmes you really want to watch and scrap the rest. Don't record them on

videotape either – all this does is shift the hour you've just saved and plonked it into another busy day, making it busier. You've just got to give something up.

4. Look at your diary and mark out the times when you are scheduled to do something else. Now strike out a couple of slots as unavailable for anything else but some form of exercise. It could be the gym, it might be sports or just time for a walk up the hill. But make it a date, not just a pencilled-in 'maybe'.

5. Decide which friends you really want to see and which you're simply hanging out with for the sake of it. Streamline your social activities so you get the most out of them, but scrap the ones which are simply stealing your time.

6. Employ the three Ds: defer; delegate, delete. There's always something you could defer to another day, ask someone else to do it or get rid of altogether. Do it now.

7. Don't commit to too much at first, otherwise it will look too daunting. Start with 2–3 sessions a week and build up. This way you'll always be successful, as opposed to promising yourself five sessions and only managing three. After a month you can add on another session.

8. Remember that formal exercise has only one purpose. By combining activity with a task you kill two birds with one stone. Examples are, car washing, window cleaning and so on. It's so much more satisfying to exercise if there's a point to it, and this type of fitness is ideal if you either hate exercise, live too far from a gym or don't like going out on your own at night.

9. Don't rely on your fitness sessions to do all the work for you. Four or five hours a week is commendable, but many women spend this amount of time every day doing

chores, walking to the shops, hand washing, etc. Add to your fitness in subtle ways.

People say they've no time to exercise, but exercise isn't something you have to slot in or make room for – it should simply be there as a normal part of life.

## Can I Reclaim my Lost Muscles?

The most comforting fact is that muscles, even after a long period of inactivity, will still regain their power if exercised again. You might feel a small grumble of stiffness but you can only get better. Tales of disaster and caution put many people off exercise when it is far more likely that you will feel youthful and energized. You can claim your 'lost' muscles; they're still there. Give them some attention and they will pay you back handsomely in terms of good looks. Remember – exercise is good for you. It is the cornerstone of successful living.

Your body might not be the shape you want it to be right now, but it can be. You have only one problem which you can't change, such as being 5ft 10in when you're 5ft 3in but the rest can be worked for. If your body doesn't seem to behave itself when you work out, challenge it a bit more. Having a great shape means working muscles to the point where they have to change shape and this is called body sculpting. They have to do it as long as you work them correctly, and this doesn't mean long hours of training – it simply means using progressively heavier weights. You can't do it overnight, but once you've got the hang of it and you're in a programme, you'll only spend twenty minutes on that body part twice a week.

## Common Myths

- 'Exercise doesn't work – I train for six hours a week and nothing's happened' – ah, but what are you doing for the other 162 hours? Exercise DOES work, but you need to be generally active as well.
- 'People who exercise are usually the ones hobbling about with injuries.' Nonsense, injuries can get better quickly. Damage to your body through disuse or lack of exercise is usually chronic and permanent.

So plan to make exercise a firm feature in your life, and get ready for the body you never thought you'd have!

## Exercise and Your Heart

Like all muscles, your heart needs exercise. By being made to work, it makes your circulation work more efficiently so it can cope with extra demand if it has to. This improves the efficiency of your legs, chest and diaphragm, and it slows your heart rate. So how much exercise is enough? Consultant cardiologist Colin Reid says, 'Three times a week at least, and you must exercise to the point of breathlessness to get any benefit. It is definitely worth it. The whole point is to build up a reserve, to cope with physical stress.'

## Exercise and Appetite

If your desire to eat was only driven by hunger, then exercise would be futile – like filling a bath with the plug out. It is thought that exercise produces an energy deficit which then increases your appetite which in turn means an increased need for food – or does it? Does energy expenditure actually increase the need to eat?

In one study, it was shown that in four groups of volunteers, the sedentary, a low-activity group, a medium-level activity group and a very active group, the sedentary group had the greatest desire to eat. Next came the very active group. Although extremely strenuous exercise usually dampens down appetite for the first twenty minutes after the activity has stopped, this group tended to reward themselves after exercise by taking their favourite foods, alcohol or a bigger meal than usual. The medium-level activity group rated third and tended to be in a reasonable energy balance, sometimes feeling that they overate, but not to a point which worried them, and finally the low-activity volunteers showed the steadiest patterns of eating. 'Low activity' was rated as the active older person, the housewife whose children have gained independence or the junior clerical worker who is basically sedentary, but active in general office duties like going to the bank, making the coffee and so on. It would seem to make sense that if the very active have a massive need to re-stock their energy supplies, then the sedentary individual would have no appetite, but we know this isn't the case. The model of the schoolgirl or the travelling account executive spring to mind, and they can in fact be the most obese of any group. They might blame it on lack of exercise, but if they have used so few calories, why the need to re-stock with so many? What is it that has driven their appetite for food?

We all know that the vast amount of eating happens for these reasons:

- Displacement activity – boredom, frustration.
- Habit food being placed before them – biscuits with coffee, etc.
- Monthly cycle – craving for food which is hormone led.
- Social environment – business lunches, hospitality, etc.
- Stress – eating which is driven by hormone release.

Once again stress comes into the picture, and think of

the two biggest appetite groups. Being very active causes adrenalin release, as does the stress of high position, the pressure of business or exams or grandchildren. The reasonably active person might not be as pressured, preferring a life where he or she is paid for the job, not the responsibility.

Boredom is also a pressure. Boredom is not necessarily doing nothing, whiling away the time, yawning, being fed-up or lonely. Boredom can be an active state. You can be rushed off your feet with the same routine day-to-day shopping, cleaning and cooking, or poring over accounts, dealing with the public, driving thousands of miles. Boredom is a bigger picture. Boredom can take over your life until you want to scream, except you reach for food instead. So this is where the low- or medium-activity person scores highest on the weight-control graph. Keeping reasonably active and eating sufficient amounts of food all lead to an energy balance, and energy balance as you know, leads to weight stability.

So does this mean that the pressured, high-status individual eats too much and can't control her weight? Of course not. The relationship between activity and hunger can take many forms, and of course the psychological status of the individual is key. Dancers are a good example. They need to be light and have low body fat, whereas the transatlantic swimmer needs to start off with rather too much fat in order to keep up with the massive energy expenditure he needs for his journey. The dancer might get extremely hungry but ignore or put off any desire to eat. Sports people are well-known for being psychologically robust in their eating and exercise discipline because there's a purpose. Being lightweight for a jockey is the difference between paying the mortgage and being broke. Even I know that if you spend your life writing about diet and fitness you have to be a reasonable example of what you preach, and I once knew a very obese man who placed a £50 bet at 20:1 that he could lose 63kg in a year – he won of course because he had that motivation behind him to make sure he didn't give up, but in general you need a goal, reason or purpose – call it what you will.

## The Psychological Benefits of Exercise

We have all heard about the benefits of exercise on our mental health and well being, and it's true. I have rarely met anybody who was bamboozled into a brisk walk and regretted it. Yes, you can get chilled to the marrow or wet or find it further than you thought it was going to be, but once home and dry, people tend to feel better for it. However, there is no single quantification of exercise which could be said to bring about mental health benefits, and the old idea of exercise being some kind of prescription has been re-examined in recent times. I think there are two factors at work here, the obvious one of fresh air, daylight and a circulation boost being naturally mood-enhancing, and the pleased-with-yourself factor. Rather like someone on a diet who manages to get through a special-occasion meal without giving in to temptation, she is pleased not disappointed with herself. Feeling strong rather than weak, as long as it is not as a result of stressfully forcing yourself to exercise, is always a positive psychological booster. However, I feel that this applies to the 'brisk walk' element of exercise or activity of the car-washing, window-cleaning type, rather than an aerobics class.

## Exercise and Endorphins

Exercise certainly boosts your 'feel good' factor by the release of chemicals called endorphins into your brain.

Endorphins are released to mask signs of pain, although you wouldn't get an endorphin release if you cut your finger. They specialize in the physical pain on exertion such as you might experience during a marathon or other endurance event, and it used to be thought that exercise addiction was due to a dependence on the effects of these chemicals, and withdrawal was caused by a period away from training or the individual's aerobics classes. However, according to Professor Clyde Williams of Loughborough University, this theory is unsound. 'If endorphins were present in everybody who was exercising at peak level, all athletes would report feeling wonderful at the end of competition – which they most certainly don't. Many athletes feel absolutely terrible, and they continue to feel terrible for another twenty-four hours, not wanting to run or race again. I'd say that the evidence for an endorphin effect is questionable.'

So what causes this 'high' which many women experience after their classes or training? I have known many scores of exercise addicts in my time, and although I have the scantiest of evidence for this theory, beyond a few dropped hints by the people concerned and my own sixth sense, I believe they all suffer from some kind of complex relationship with food and weight. Exercise is the means by which these individuals can control their eating and body shape, and when exercise is not possible they suffer mental torment. In fact, I clearly remember an occasion when I used to teach fitness classes, when the caretaker of one of my premises failed to turn up to unlock. After a long wait I decided to abandon the class, only to turn round to the assembled throng in the car park to see several women crying. I asked what was wrong. 'I always have a cake after lunch on Tuesday,' said one, 'because I know I've got my class later on. I just don't know what I'm going to do now.'

To a woman who relies on exercise, life is stressful. To be able to complete her exercise schedule or even to exceed it is to be relieved of stress, and it is this sensation that causes her joy and happiness. Yes, endorphins undoubtedly exist and many people experience them. They are also released at other times such as during the cold shower or the terrifying fairground ride, but when it comes to the story of your brain and its effect on your attitudes to exercise, endorphins are only part of a complex story.

## Insulin Sensitivity

Exercise improves insulin sensitivity which helps to lose fat, particularly in the central part of your body. Training can reduce abdominal fat and increase the size and tone of the gluteus muscle in your buttocks, hence helping to raise your metabolism. Experts agree that this reduced-sugar diet should be recommended before the menopause sets in (in your mid-thirties), before the fat is already laid down. On the dietary front, it has been found recently that linoleic acid found in sunflower oil improves insulin sensitivity, thereby reducing the central adiposity (fat).

## Starting Young

A lot of the problems happen at school and are laid at the door of competitive sports. Sports allow the talented to shine, but they can produce feelings of inadequacy and inferiority in people either less well endowed or with poor coordination. Some of the confusion in this debate has come about because exercise is a vague word which conjures up a variety of muscle-building endurance feats. Young children are naturally active, but by the time they start school social development can hinder participation in sports. If your teenager shies away from games at school, this is what they should be doing:

- Joint Mobility: your body should be able to function as it was built, so joints should be put through their full range of movement daily. Arm circling, leg swinging, ankle flexing, toe touching, etc.
- Bone Loading: your bones need loading to provide strength and density. All weight-bearing exercise is important, such as running and walking. If you sit in front of a TV or computer all the time, you risk postural and bone-weakening problems.
- Endurance: anyone aged between twelve and nineteen should have the capacity to take part in sport, run and climb without any severe exhaustion, pain or breathlessness. If you are worried that you are getting fat, rather than sit and worry, why not consider getting a dog which needs walking? If you've already got one, do you take it out or does someone else? Do it yourself! Also offer to do the shopping and walk back with laden bags.

## Exercise in Your Teens

From as early as twelve or thirteen, exercise should start to concentrate on strength training, and for this a young teenager would use her own bodyweight as resistance. Examples of good exercises are press-ups, chin-ups and handstands to develop a good firm bustline and arms, with hill cycling and swimming for shapely legs and buttocks. Actual weight-training is not a good idea just yet because growth cartilage can be easily damaged, but this is only a worry if you are training too hard as a competitive sports-woman or gymnast. At all stages of life but particularly now, bone strengthening, muscle development and cardio-vascular endurance can only be good for your body and shape. Stretching also improves posture, which will make the most of your figure, lending a leaner, longer look to your entire body. Go for an eight-week programme to get you started, doing just two strength sessions a week. Daily walking of no less than forty-five minutes is a must too. One of the main benefits will be less painful periods and a relief from premenstrual symptoms.

## Exercise in Your Twenties and Thirties

Your exercise at this age should start to concentrate on muscle development and maintenance, because poor muscles at this stage are harder to regain later on. You should aim for at least four dedicated exercise sessions every week, even if these are done at home. My mini-books *Monica's Fabulous Body Plans* for four body areas: thighs; bottoms; midriffs and abdominals; bust, arms and backs, all have complete exercise programmes in them, giving full instructions, right down to when you stand up and lie down again! They each include a home-based plan for which you need absolutely no equipment or facilities other than a flight of stairs and a standard doorstep.

## Exercise and Pregnancy

Being pregnant doesn't mean you have to get out of shape. Here are a few tips for a healthy nine months:

- If you are planning to get pregnant, strengthen your abdominal muscles first. Exercise on alternate days with curl-ups and back strengthening exercises.
- Until the fourth month, do daily mobility exercises for your joints, plus gentle abdominal toning.
- Do 5 minutes on an exercise bike, followed by stretching, then 20 minutes of cycling or water aerobics or very low impact aerobics. Cool down slowly.
- After the fourth month, avoid exercises lying on your back. Sleep on your side.

- After the fifth month take care with stretching. The hormonal changes cause ligament softening which can lead to tears and injury. Do standing pelvic tilts and squeezes.
- After the birth wait until your post-natal all-clear before starting exercise again. Build up slowly, starting with daily walks, cycling and three minutes of stomach exercises, to a total of three hours a week. Add half an hour a fortnight until you are doing five hours a week apart from general activity.

## Stopping the Clock

The thirties are when the first age-related fitness problems start to rear their heads. Physiotherapist Clair Flynn deals with many sports injuries in her clinic. 'Muscle starts to be lost from the age of thirty,' she says. 'Joint lubrication suffers, and this is an age when people start to gain a little weight through slower metabolism and they tend to get more competitive at games. The muscles aren't up to it and they get injured.' Other common problems in the thirties are:

- spinal and sports injuries
- problems from sitting too long
- injuries from carrying small children
- repetitive strain injuries
- problems caused by work stations
- injuries caused by driving
- obesity damage to hips and knees

The biggest problem, says Clair Flynn, is long-distance driving. She recommends that if you drive more than 500 miles a week you should stop every hour to walk around and stretch – this keeps your spine mobile.

I have my own tip for drivers, and that is when you stop at motorway services, park as far away from the front entrance as you can, and walk quickly or run to the building. It might be only a short distance each way but it is better than parking a few metres away. Remember the accumulation factor: do this a few times a month and you're clocking up calories used!

## Exercise in Your Forties and Fifties

The only difference you need to be aware of in your midlife is the effect of hormones on ligaments, and this is why even if you were one of the founder members of the aerobics generation, you need to be aware of particularly strong stretches and major effort through the body, much as you would get on a long uphill cycle ride. Pushing hard through the spine as you do when bearing down on pedals or when uphill walking or climbing, can be felt in your lower back a little more in your forties and fifties simply because the hormonal effects on your pelvic region and back make for congestion, water retention and soft ligaments – rather like the soft ligaments of pregnancy. You can gain weight quite easily at this age, but there again you can gain weight at any age. 'Middle-age spread' is not inevitable. You should anticipate these changes by using progressively heavier weights in simple routines – there's no need to go mad. Two, twenty-minute sessions a week for upper body and two for lower body will be enough to keep you in tip-top shape well into your sixties and seventies.

## Your Plan of Action

1. Exercise aerobically for forty-five minutes on alternate days. You should be breathless.

2. In your teens, add resistance work and swimming.

3. In your twenties and thirties, add yoga, Pilates and weights.

4. In your midlife and beyond, concentrate on weights, swimming and yoga.

## To Conclude

Exercise is brilliant for your hormones, and it is known that women who exercise regularly, or who lead an active, industrious life, have far fewer hormone problems than those who don't. This is not just coincidence. Your body is made to do a variety of movements, your insulin is there to regulate the blood sugars which are 'exercised' when you are aerobically active, and your female hormones are affected by the amount of fat on your body. It always makes sense to exercise and as long as you do the right exercise, you don't stress yourself by overdoing it and you get enough rest your body chaos can only benefit from exercise. Indeed, I have known clients of mine, previously true couch potatoes, who have banished all their period pains, anxiety, depression and hot flushes simply by exercising aerobically four times a week.

So get to love exercise! Your body will pay you back many times in terms of shape and body contentment.

# Chapter Eleven

# Recipes

## Apricot and Almond Flapjack

**Makes 12 pieces. Calories per piece: 180.**

This delicious flapjack takes minutes to make. It's not too sweet, but if you have a piece when you feel your energy levels falling and an urge to head for the chocolate, it removes those cravings totally! I always have a piece at 4 o'clock in the afternoon when it seems a long time since lunch. You can add other ingredients like sultanas or sunflower seeds according to taste.

---

| | |
|---|---|
| 200g dried apricots, chopped | ½ tsp cinnamon |
| 100g Olivio | 1 tbsp sesame seeds |
| 100g sugar-free apricot and peach jam | 200g porridge oats |
| 50g toasted flaked almonds, roughly crushed by hand | |

---

Pre-heat the oven to 180°C/375°F/gas mark 5.

Put all the ingredients except the oats into a large heavy pan and heat through gently until the Olivio has melted. Turn up the heat and simmer gently for five minutes, stirring all the time. Take off the heat and stir in the oats, combining well.

Press the mixture into a square dish, or baking sheet, to a depth of an inch and bake in a moderate oven for 20–30 minutes. Leave to cool in the tin, but slice into about 12 squares very carefully first – you might need to use a slightly damp knife. Remove when completely cold, and store in an airtight container. Wrap individual slices to take out with you.

## Apricot and Brazil Nut Bread

Makes one large loaf. Calories per slice: approx. 90, depending on thickness.

| | |
|---|---|
| 500g strong white bread flour | ½ tsp cinnamon |
| 1½ tsp salt | 280 ml tepid water |
| 1½ tsp dried yeast | 12 brazil nuts, flaked |
| 1 tbsp sugar | 200g chopped apricots |
| 1 tbsp walnut oil | |

Sift the flour into a large bowl and add the salt, yeast, sugar, oil and cinnamon. Make a well in the centre and add 280 ml tepid water. Mix together gently but thoroughly until it begins to form into a ball.

Turn onto a floured board and knead gently for no less than ten minutes. Sprinkle the nuts and apricots over the dough and press them into the dough lightly. Knead well for another 2 minutes to incorporate them.

Put the dough into a floured bowl, cover with a damp cloth or clingfilm and leave in a warm but not hot place to rise. It should take about an hour to an hour and a half for the dough to have doubled in size. Remove from bowl and 'knock back' by pressing all the air out of the dough for a minute. Shape into a ball and put the dough either into a large well-greased and floured loaf tin or divide in two and use two smaller tins.

Cover and allow to rise for a further hour or so.

Pre-heat the oven to 230°C/450°F/gas mark 8 and put the

bread to cook in the centre of the hot oven for about 15–20 minutes according to the size of loaf. Test that the loaf is ready by gently removing from the tin and tapping the base which should sound hollow if it's cooked. Remove immediately and cool on a wire rack.

## Banana Cake

Makes 12 slices. Calories per slice: 110.

| | |
|---|---|
| 175g Olivio | 2 ripe bananas, thinly sliced |
| 120g caster sugar | 2–3 drops banana essence |
| 2 eggs | 175–225g self-raising flour, sifted |

Pre-heat the oven to 180°C/350°F/gas mark 4.

Grease or line a 500g loaf tin.

Beat the Olivio with the sugar until pale and creamy and add the eggs one at a time. Add the bananas and 2–3 drops of banana essence (be careful, it's strong). Fold in the sifted flour and turn the whole mixture into the loaf tin, slightly hollowing the centre of the cake.

Bake for 45–60 minutes, remembering to test the centre of the cake with a fork to make sure it's done. Turn onto a wire rack to cool and remove the lining paper.

Serve in slices as a meal break, or with fresh fruit salad.

## Banana and Tofu Cream Dessert

Makes about 4 portions. Calories per portion: 110.

| | |
|---|---|
| 1 large banana | 50g ground almonds |
| 100g tofu | 1 tbsp natural yoghurt |

Simply put all the ingredients into a blender, or use a hand blender (the mixture tends to be a little stiff) and blend thoroughly, divide into small pots and refrigerate.

## Beef Bourguignonne

Serves 4. Calories per serving: about 300 (minus the vegetables).

This dish is extremely low in fat, but high in protein, vitamin B12 and iron. It is good served with either rice or small new potatoes, and crisp green vegetables.

| | |
|---|---|
| 1 dsp vegetable oil | 4 dsp tomato puree |
| 1 onion, sliced | 6 rashers best smoked back bacon, cut |
| 700g best lean stewing or braising steak | into 2cm strips |
| (such as Aberdeen Angus), cubed | 50g baby mushrooms |
| 2 standard glasses any red wine | mixed fresh herbs |
| ½ clove garlic, crushed (optional) | 2 tbsp half-fat crème fraiche |
| salt and black pepper | fresh parsley (preferably flat-leaved), |
| 2 tins standard supermarket range chopped | coarsely chopped |
| tomatoes with added herbs and olives | |

Pre-heat the oven to 160°C/325°F/gas mark 3.

Heat the oil in a large pan, and add the sliced onion. Keeping the heat moderate, turn the onion constantly for a few minutes, until it is transparent.

Add the cubed beef. Keep turning to seal all sides, until all traces of red have gone. Then add the wine, crushed garlic,

2 glasses of plain water and season. Stir well.

Transfer the contents of the pan to a casserole dish, put the lid on tightly, and place in oven for 1½ hours.

Remove from oven, and add the tinned tomatoes, tomato puree and the bacon strips. Stir well. Return to oven for a further hour.

Take the casserole out of the oven and stir well. Add a little more water if needed, although the casserole should not be too wet by now. Add the whole baby mushrooms and check the seasoning and add a sprinkling of mixed herbs, to taste. Return to oven to heat through.

Just before serving, stir in 2 tbsp half-fat crème fraiche, and top with a good sprinkling of coarsely chopped fresh parsley.

## Carrot and Orange Cake

Makes 10–12 slices. Calories per slice: 140.

| | |
|---|---|
| 120g Olivio | juice of 1½ oranges |
| 60g sugar | 120–175g self-raising flour |
| 2 eggs | 2 drops vanilla essence |
| 120g carrots, grated | pinch mixed spice |
| grated rind of two large oranges | |

Pre-heat the oven to 180°C/350°F/gas mark 4. Line a 500g loaf tin with non-stick baking parchment.

Cream the Olivio and sugar together until creamy then add the eggs and, using an electric beater, beat until pale. Add the grated carrots, orange rind and juice, then fold in the flour. Add two drops of vanilla essence and a pinch of mixed spice. Pour into the loaf tin and bake in the centre of the oven for about 45 minutes.

## Cheese and Potato Pie

Serves 4. Calories per serving: 455.

---

| | |
|---|---|
| 1 onion, chopped finely and fried gently in 1 tbsp oil | 2–3 teacups semi-skimmed milk |
| | 120g strong Cheddar cheese |
| 4 × large potatoes, boiled and cubed | salt and pepper |
| 4 carrots, boiled and chopped | fresh parsley |
| 1 tbsp cornflour | |

---

Pre-heat the oven to 200°C/400°F/gas mark 6.

Put the onion, half the potatoes and all the carrots into a plastic bag, add the cornflour, and shake very gently to coat. Turn them out into an ovenproof dish and pour the milk over them. Stir gently to incorporate the cornflour. Season well and stir in the parsley.

Mash the remaining potatoes, cover the top of the pie with the mash and top with all the grated cheese.

Put into the medium hot oven for about 20 minutes. Grill the top if desired, to make a golden crunchy topping.

## Date and Walnut Cake

Makes 10–12 slices. Calories per slice: 165.

---

| | |
|---|---|
| 225g dates | 120g walnuts |
| 90g sugar | 120g Olivio |
| 150ml water | 225g self-raising flour |
| 1 tsp bicarbonate of soda | 3 eggs |

---

Pre-heat the oven to 180°C/350°F/gas mark 4. Line a 500g loaf tin with non-stick parchment paper or greaseproof paper.

Put the dates, sugar and water in a pan over a medium heat, bring to a gentle simmer and leave to cook for about

5–10 minutes. The dates and water should have become a soft sauce-like mixture. Remove from the heat and add the bicarbonate of soda, walnuts and Olivio, allow to cool.

Fold in the flour and beaten eggs. Pour into the loaf tin and cook in the centre of the oven for about 45 minutes.

## Fruit Yoghurts

Calories per pot: approx. 150.

This is simply an easy way to make your own fruited yoghurt without all those additives, and it gives you a low GI filler or dessert to keep you energized for 2–3 hours. They are low in fat, high in potassium, calcium and protein. You will find these yoghurts very calming for the nerves.

### Banana Yoghurt
Take a 150g pot bio or soya yoghurt and mix in half a chopped banana, 1 tsp ground almonds. Put a pinch of cinnamon on top.

### Apricot Yoghurt
Take a 150g pot bio or soya yoghurt and mix in 6 chopped dried apricots and 15g flaked almonds.

### Rhubarb Yoghurt
Take a 150g pot bio or soya yoghurt and mix in 1 large tbsp tinned rhubarb in natural juice, 1 tsp Froment and a pinch of ginger.

### Ginger and Raisin Yoghurt
Take a 150g pot of bio or soya yoghurt and mix in 2 chopped stems of crystallized ginger and 2 tsp raisins.

### Fresh Berry Yoghurt
Take a 150g pot of bio or soya yoghurt and mix in 3 sliced strawberries, 1 dsp blueberries, a few raspberries and mango

chunks. Turn into small bowl and top with 1 tsp Froment and 1 tsp roughly chopped hazelnuts.

### Fruit and Nut Yoghurt

Take a 150g pot of bio or soya yoghurt and mix in 1 tsp toasted sunflower seeds, 1 tsp toasted pine kernels, 1 tsp toasted sesame seeds, 6 sliced fresh green grapes.

## Winter Fruit Salad

Calories per tablespoon: approx 80.

| | |
|---|---|
| tin of prunes in apple juice | 6 tinned figs |
| 12 dried apricots | 1 banana, sliced |
| 60g flaked almonds (optional) | |

Put all the ingredients together in a large bowl, making sure the banana is covered by the juice. Store in the fridge and use for breakfast, pudding or as a topping for yoghurt.

## Grilled Chicken in Orange Marinade

Serves 1. Calories per serving: 210

| | |
|---|---|
| 150–200g skinless, boneless chicken breast | 1 tbsp walnut oil (or olive oil) |
| | clove garlic (optional) |
| juice and rind of 1 large orange | |

Place all the ingredients in an ovenproof dish, stir well to mix, cover with foil and refrigerate overnight if possible, for a whole day or a minimum of two hours.

Pre-heat the oven to 180°C/350°F/gas mark 4. Remove the chicken from the dish and place on a wire rack over a roasting tin in the oven. Cook for about 20 minutes.

Turn the grill to high, and finish off the chicken by grilling thoroughly on both sides until brown and slightly caramelized.

Alternatively pan-fry with the lid on tightly, over medium heat, turning frequently to prevent burning. This takes about 10 minutes.

## Lentil Soup

Makes 8 × 250ml bowls. Calories per serving: approx. 200.

The beauty of this incredibly nutritious, filling soup is the ease with which you make it, the fact that it fills you like no other soup can, and that it is positively bursting with goodness. Make a quantity on a Sunday to see you through the week.

| | |
|---|---|
| 200g red lentils | 2 medium turnips, peeled and chopped |
| small pat butter | 2 sticks celery, washed and chopped |
| 1 large onion, peeled and sliced | salt and black pepper |
| 4 large rashers smoked back bacon (optional) | celery salt (optional) |
| | little single cream (optional) |
| 6 large carrots, peeled and chopped | fresh parsley, chopped |

Soak the lentils in water overnight. Drain well.

Put the butter into a large pan, add the onion and bacon and sauté slowly until the onion is transparent. Add the chopped carrots, turnips, celery, lentils and enough water to cover the vegetables. Leave to simmer very gently for about 45 minutes.

Take off the heat and allow to cool a little. Discard the bacon completely. Pour everything into a blender or food processor (or rub through a sieve). Process for a few seconds, or until at the consistency you prefer.

Put back in the saucepan and add salt and pepper to taste, and a little extra celery salt if desired.

Add a little swirl of light cream on the top, if you like, and a good sprinkling of chopped parsley. Serve with crusty granary or wholemeal bread.

## Liver with Dubonnet and Orange

Serves 2. Calories per serving: 325.

| For the liver | For the sauce |
|---|---|
| 1 tbsp oil | 1 tbsp (heaped) plain flour, seasoned |
| ½ onion, finely chopped | grated rind and juice of 2 oranges |
| 1 tbsp flour mixed with salt and pepper | 1 wine glass Dubonnet |
| 350g lamb's liver, sliced | handful chopped fresh parsley |

Heat the oil in a large frying-pan, add the onion and fry gently for 5 minutes.

Put the flour, salt and pepper into a plastic bag, add the sliced liver and shake thoroughly. Remove and shake off excess flour.

Add to the pan, fry gently for a few minutes, turning once. Arrange the liver on a serving dish and surround with either rice or mashed potato. Keep warm.

For the sauce, add the flour to the remains of the juices in the pan and stir to get rid of any lumps. Tip the orange juice and rind into the pan and stir. Take off the heat and add the Dubonnet. Pour over the liver and garnish with parsley.

## Main Meal Salad

Serves 1. Calories per serving: approx. 38.

This main meal salad has an abundance of vitamins, minerals, water, protein and carbohydrates. Have it on its own, or as an accompaniment to chicken, salmon or tofu.

| | |
|---|---|
| lettuce | 1 tbsp cooked beetroot, grated |
| watercress | chicory |
| cucumber, sliced | ½ stick celery |
| mustard and cress | shredded white or red cabbage |
| rocket | 1 tbsp cooked peas, cooled |
| lambs lettuce | ½ avocado, sliced |
| sliced tomato | 1 rasher back bacon, well grilled, chopped |
| 1 tbsp sweetcorn | 3–4 segments tinned pink grapefruit |
| few small florets cauliflower | 15g toasted pine kernels |
| 1 tbsp carrot, grated | 1 dsp oil and vinegar dressing |
| rings of coloured pepper | |

Combine all the ingredients in a bowl and pour over the dressing.

## Meatballs in Tomato Sauce

Makes enough for 2–3 portions. Calories per serving: 220.

| | |
|---|---|
| 450g leanest mince | garlic *or* onions and peppers (available from supermarkets) |
| 3–4 slices stale white bread, in breadcrumbs | 2 tbsp tomato paste |
| salt and black pepper | sprinkling mixed herbs |
| 1 egg, beaten | chopped parsley |
| 2 tins chopped tomatoes with onions and | |

Put the meat into a bowl. Add the breadcrumbs, salt and

black pepper (to taste), and the beaten egg. Using your hands, mix the whole thing together, then take out small handfuls and form into balls. Tip the tins of tomatoes, the tomato paste and the mixed herbs into a large, ovenproof dish and stir. Add the meatballs to the tomato mixture. Cover the dish with foil, and bake in a medium oven, 180°C/350°F/gas mark 4, for an hour.

Take off the foil for the last 20 minutes of cooking time and spoon the sauce over the meatballs. Return to the oven so that the meat browns.

Serve with rice or spaghetti. The Scandinavian way would be to serve on a bed of mashed potato, with fresh peas. Sprinkle with parsley before serving.

## Mixed Cooked Salad

This makes enough for 4 portions. Calories per portion: 120.

| For the salad | For the dressing |
|---|---|
| 4 tbsp cooked peas | 1 tbsp fresh mayonnaise |
| 4 tbsp sweetcorn | 1 tbsp half-fat crème fraiche |
| 4 tbsp diced beetroot | few fronds snipped fresh dill or 1–2 tsp |
| 4 carrots, chopped into matchsticks, | dried dill |
| steamed and cooled | black pepper |
| 1 medium potato, boiled, cooled and diced | |

Simply put all the salad ingredients into a bowl. Combine all the dressing ingredients in another bowl. Then mix the two together. Put into a container with a lid and refrigerate. Best eaten with cold meat or fish.

## Pasta with Green Vegetable Sauce

Serves 2–3 depending on whether eaten as a light or a main meal.
Calories per serving: 270.

---

2 teacups dried pasta shapes (about
   150g weight before cooking)

100g broad beans, boiled and cooled

100g fresh peas, boiled and cooled

12 asparagus tips (optional, and tinned
   will do)

1 courgette, sliced, with skin on

2 tbsp walnut or sunflower oil

2 large tbsp half-fat crème fraiche

½ tsp dried tarragon or few chopped fresh
   tarragon leaves

salt and black pepper

bunch fresh parsley, chopped

few shavings fresh Parmesan (to taste)

---

Boil the pasta according to directions on the packet. Drain
and reserve.

While the pasta is cooking stir-fry all the vegetables in the
oil for about 2–3 minutes in a large frying pan. Make sure
you slightly sear the courgette and asparagus. Add the
cooked pasta shapes and mix together to heat through. Add
the crème fraiche and, keeping on a low heat, stir through to
heat gently without curdling. Finally, add the herbs and
season.

Turn out onto hot plates (pasta gets cold very quickly),
top with the parsley and add Parmesan to taste.


## Simple Gooseberry Fool

Serves 4. Calories per serving: 165

---

900g gooseberries

4 tbsp caster sugar

6 artificial tablet sweeteners

300ml (2 pots) plain bio yoghurt

4 tbsp half-fat crème fraiche

---

Pick over the gooseberries to get rid of stalks and wash
thoroughly. Place them in a heavy-bottomed pan with the

sugar, crush a few gooseberries to release the juice and let them steam without adding any other liquid until soft. Stir in the sweeteners. Leave them to cool.

Meanwhile, in a bowl stir the yoghurt and crème fraiche together then fold in the gooseberry mixture. Spoon into individual pots or small ramekin dishes and, if eating formally rather than as a quick lunch at work, garnish with a few whole, stewed gooseberries.

This can also be made with blackcurrants, strawberries, raspberries or cherries.


## Spanish Omelette

Serves 1. Calories per serving: 250.

| | |
|---|---|
| ¼ onion, finely chopped and sautéed in 1 dsp oil, cool | 3 large eggs |
| 1 dsp vegetable oil | salt and black pepper |
| 3 rings each red and yellow pepper | a few shavings of Parmesan cheese (optional) |
| 1 small potato, boiled and cubed | 1 tbsp fresh parsley, chopped |
| 1 tbsp French or runner beans, chopped | |

Put the onion back into the frying-pan, add another dsp oil and add all the other vegetables. Fry through very gently.

Whisk the eggs together with salt and black pepper and when the vegetables are slightly browned pour the eggs over them. Heat through without turning for about 3–4 minutes, until the bottom of the omelette is cooked but the top is still runny.

Meanwhile, pre-heat the grill to high then place the frying-pan underneath. Brown the top of the omelette for a few minutes until cooked but not dry or hard.

Serve with some grated shavings of Parmesan cheese and parsley.

## Stir-fried Vegetable Curry

Serves 4. Calories per serving: about 300; with rice, 480.

This simple curry keeps the mixture 'dry', and free from heavy, fattening sauces. Serve on plain boiled rice.

| | |
|---|---|
| 250g long-grain rice | 200g cooked French beans |
| 4 tbsp walnut oil | 200g baby corn |
| ½ onion, peeled and chopped finely | 1 red and 1 yellow pepper, chopped into |
| ½ clove garlic, crushed | rings |
| 450g old potatoes, peeled, boiled, cooled and chopped | 1 small red chilli pepper, sliced finely |
| | 1 dsp standard curry powder (mild or hot, |
| 450g cooked carrots, cooled and chopped | according to taste) |
| 200g cooked peas | fresh parsley, chopped |

Cook the rice according to the instructions on the packet.

Heat the oil in a large heavy-based frying pan. Add the chopped onion and crushed garlic, and fry gently until soft. Then add all the vegetables, turning well to coat with the oil. Add a little more oil if the mixture looks dry or is in danger of burning. Heat through for about 3 minutes. Add the curry powder, turning quickly to coat all the vegetables. Add a little more to taste if necessary.

Turn out over rice, onto hot plates, measuring 4 tbsp rice per person. Sprinkle with parsley and eat at once.

## Spiced Rice Pudding with Sultanas

Makes about 8 small pots. Calories per pot: 140.

| | |
|---|---|
| 2.2 litres semi-skimmed milk | 6 artificial sweeteners |
| 120g organic brown pudding rice | 100g largest possible sultanas |
| 2 tbsp sugar | fresh grated nutmeg |
| ½ to 1 tsp cinnamon to taste | |

Pre-heat the oven to 160°C/325°F/gas mark 3.

Bring the milk to the boil in a pan, or heat through for about 10 minutes in the microwave.

Put the rice, sugar and cinnamon in a large ovenproof basin and pour the milk over them, stirring well to prevent the rice sticking together. Place in a medium to low oven for 2 hours, stirring regularly.

When the rice is cooked, remove and add the sweeteners and sultanas. Stir well to incorporate. Grate nutmeg on the top.

Cool, then divide into individual pots, ramekins or clean, washed yoghurt pots.

Cover and refrigerate until needed.

## Sweet Marscapone Mousse

Serves 8. Calories per serving: 280.

| | |
|---|---|
| 450g Marscapone cheese | 400g frozen summer fruits, such as |
| 4 egg whites | redcurrants, raspberries, blueberries, etc. |
| 75g caster sugar | small amaretto biscuits (optional) to serve |

Put the Marscapone cheese into a mixing bowl and, using a wooden spoon, beat until smooth.

Put the egg whites into a clean bowl and whip with an electric whisk for 30 seconds or until fairly stiff. Add half the sugar; whip again, then the rest of the sugar. Whip on high speed until quite stiff but not dry. Fold into the cheese then chill for about an hour.

Next, put a layer of the marscapone mousse into individual serving dishes, then add a layer of berries, and repeat until you have about 4–5 layers.

To serve, top with a sprig of redcurrants and dust with icing sugar.

## Thai Turkey Salad

Serves 4. Calories per serving: about 265.

This warm salad seems to be a fiddle to make when you look at the list of marinade ingredients, but in fact it is incredibly simple. Things like lemon grass, ginger fish sauce and chilli oil can be bought in reasonable amounts and last in the fridge for weeks enabling you to make this dish, or variations of it, many times. You can also use beef, lamb, tofu or Quorn instead of turkey to ring the changes. It really is worth the effort!

**For the marinade**

2 stalks lemon grass, finely chopped

5cm piece root ginger, peeled and finely chopped

2 shallots, finely chopped

2 cloves garlic, crushed

juice of 2 limes

4 tbsp soft brown sugar

2 tsp fish sauce

2 tbsp chilli oil

**For the turkey**

450g turkey breast fillets, sliced into long, thin strips

2 tbsp vegetable oil

**For the salad**

275g Chinese cabbage, shredded finely

175g cucumber, cut into long thin strips

175g water chestnuts, sliced

1 fresh red chilli, cut in rings

1 carrot, peeled and chopped into matchstick lengths

handful of fresh coriander, chopped

**For the dressing**

2 tbsp fish sauce

2 tbsp wine vinegar

2 tbsp vegetable oil

handful of fresh coriander, chopped

pinch sugar

Place the marinade ingredients in a bowl and mix together. Add the sliced turkey to the marinade and mix well. Refrigerate overnight if possible, or for 1 hour at least.

Put the Chinese leaves, cucumber, water chestnuts, chilli pepper, carrot and coriander in a serving bowl.

Place the dressing ingredients into a screw-topped jar and shake together well.

Heat a little oil, in a large frying pan and add the strips of turkey carefully. Fry over a medium heat for about 5 minutes, turning constantly. Test that the turkey is cooked through by cutting into a strip – it should be white throughout.

To serve, pour a little of the dressing over the raw salad, mix, add the hot turkey and divide between the four plates. Eat immediately.

## Vegetable Chilli

Makes 2 portions. Calories per portion: 240.

| | |
|---|---|
| 1 teacup Basmati rice | 12 mushrooms, sliced |
| 2 tbsp vegetable oil | 1 small green chilli pepper, chopped |
| 1/4 onion, chopped finely | 6 tbsp chopped tomatoes with herbs |
| 1 clove garlic, crushed | (tinned) |
| 4 tbsp pre-cooked, tinned, red kidney | 1 tsp chilli powder (or to taste) |
| beans | salt and black pepper, to taste |
| half each, red, green and yellow pepper, | fresh parsley, roughly chopped |
| chopped finely | |

Boil the rice according to the instructions on the packet. Drain well and reserve.

In a large frying pan, put the oil, onion and garlic. Fry gently until the onion is transparent but not browned. Add the rest of the vegetables and fry through gently. Keep stirring. Add the tinned tomatoes and stir thoroughly. Stir in the chilli powder and season.

When the mixture is cooked through, re-heat the rice thoroughly, in a microwave if possible. Divide both the vegetables and the rice between two plates and garnish with freshly chopped parsley.

## Warm Chicken or Beef Salad

Serves 1. Calories per serving: 450.

This is simple: all you need to do is stir-fry 200g strips fresh chicken or fillet steak in a little oil, then season with 1 tbsp soy sauce. While still sizzling, pour straight onto a bed of fresh salad greens. Top with a French dressing made from walnut oil and balsamic vinegar.

# Finally

We're all here for such a short time that overcoming your body chaos is worth a shot. It isn't that hard. The hardest part of all is taking that first step to rediscovering yourself, but I hope I've shown you that life only ends when it ends, and it's the quality of your life that counts.

Eating well is common sense, but I understand that taking the steps towards change are like picking up the phone to someone you dread talking to, or phoning to pay a bill. You just can't bring yourself to do it: you'll do it tomorrow; you'll wait till next week; you'll ask someone else to do it for you or better still – you'll forget it. Well, you can easily sideline your body chaos because it has a habit of going away but, like those bills you can't get round to paying, they've got a habit of coming back as red reminders! So before your body gets the equivalent of the bailiffs at the door, do something. Say 'Stop!' to your old chaotic life and grab those hormones by the throat. You're going to start tomorrow, take steps and feel better than ever before. This is the only life you've got and you don't want to spend most of it in bitterness. Then one day you'll be saying to your friends, 'Oh, I used to suffer terrible hormones – but they got better all by themselves.'

Good luck.

# Food File

Basic guide to food values, calories, proteins, carbohydrates and fats.

## Carbohydrate and Sugar Guide

Choose carbohydrates which are low in added sugars. If you are trying to lose weight, take your carbohydrates from fruit, vegetables and milk, with low glycaemic index starches added when appropriate.

The grams in this guide have all been rounded up or down to the nearest whole number. It is intended as a guide only, but daily carbohydrate intake should be around 200g. Some sugars are naturally occurring, e.g. lactose, maltose, fructose, etc. Sweet products such as biscuits contain added sugars. Products such as jams contain a mixture of both.

| PRODUCT | CARBOHYDRATE (g) | SUGAR (g) |
|---|---|---|
| **BEANS, TINNED (per 100 g)** | | |
| Butter beans | 15.0 | 5.0 |
| Chilli beans | 20.0 | 5.0 |
| Baked beans in tomato sauce | 18.0 | 6.0 |
| Reduced sugar beans | 13.0 | 5.0 |

| PRODUCT | CARBOHYDRATE (g) | SUGAR (g) |
|---|---|---|
| **NON-ALCOHOLIC BEVERAGES (made according to directions)** | | |
| Drinking chocolate | 11.0 | 11.0 |
| Options Chocolate | 5.0 | 5.0 |
| Horlicks | 19.0 | 11.0 |
| Horlicks Light | 22.0 | 19.0 |
| Ovaltine Powder | 16.0 | 13.0 |
| **BISCUITS (per biscuit)** | | |
| Custard cream | 7.0 | 3.0 |
| Plain digestive | 10.0 | 3.0 |
| Chocolate digestive | 11.0 | 5.0 |
| Jaffa Cake | 9.0 | 6.0 |
| Cream crackers | 5.0 | NIL |
| Ryvita Multigrain (slice) | 6.0 | 0.2 |
| **BREAD (each)** | | |
| Baguette | 7.0 | NIL |
| Danish loaf (per slice) | 7.0 | 0.3 |
| Crumpet | 12.0 | 1.5 |
| Pitta bread | 9.0 | 0.4 |
| Naan bread | 63.2 | 14.0 |
| **BREAKFAST CEREALS (per serving)** | | |
| All Bran | 14.0 | 6.0 |
| Cornflakes | 25.0 | 3.0 |
| Coco Pops | 25.0 | 12.0 |
| Strike | 23.0 | 1.0 |
| Shredded Wheat | 26.0 | 1.0 |
| Sugar Puffs | 25.0 | 15.0 |
| Special K | 23.0 | 5.0 |
| Weetabix | 20.0 | 1.0 |

| PRODUCT | CARBOHYDRATE (g) | SUGAR (g) |
|---|---|---|
| **CAKES (each)** | | |
| Eccles cake | 27.0 | 15.0 |
| Almond slice | 15.0 | 10.0 |
| Jam Swiss roll (slice) | 28.0 | 21.0 |
| Chocolate Swiss roll (slice) | 24.0 | 17.0 |
| Rich fruit cake (slice) | 45.0 | 42.0 |
| Apple pie (individual) | 39.0 | 18.0 |
| Meringue nest | 14.0 | 14.0 |
| **CONFECTIONERY (per 100g)** | | |
| Barley sugar | 97.0 | 97.0 |
| Brazil nut toffees | 67.0 | 67.0 |
| Dolly Mixtures | 91.0 | 91.0 |
| Milk chocolate | 58.0 | 55.0 |
| Plain chocolate | 58.0 | 56.0 |
| **CRISPS AND SNACKS (per bag)** | | |
| Assorted crisps, all flavours | 12.0 | 0.3 |
| Low fat crisps | 15.0 | 0.2 |
| Potato rings | 14.0 | 0.1 |
| Tortilla chips | 23.0 | 2.0 |
| **DRINKS** | | |
| Cola | 11.0 | 11.0 |
| All diet drinks | NIL | NIL |
| Lemon crush | 10.0 | 10.0 |
| Lemonade | 6.0 | 6.0 |
| Tropical fruit crush | 13.0 | 13.0 |
| Whole orange | 9.0 | 9.0 |
| Sugar-free orange | 1.0 | 1.0 |
| Lime juice cordial | 9.0 | 9.0 |

**EGGS have no carbohydrate or sugar**

| PRODUCT | CARBOHYDRATE (g) | SUGAR (g) |
|---|---|---|
| **FATS have little carbohydrate or sugar with these exceptions** | | |
| Garlic butter | 2.0 | 0.2 |
| Healthy eating lowest ever | 6.0 | 3.0 |
| Olive oil spread | 1.0 | 1.0 |

**FISH has no carbohydrate or sugar unless coated in breadcrumbs or batter**

| **FRUIT (tinned in juice per 100g)** | | |
|---|---|---|
| Apricot halves | 10.0 | 10.0 |
| Fruit cocktail | 11.0 | 11.0 |
| Grapefruit segments | 10.0 | 10.0 |
| Prunes | 22.0 | 22.0 |
| Mandarin oranges | 8.0 | 8.0 |
| Mixed fruit | 14.0 | 14.0 |
| Orange segments | 11.0 | 11.0 |
| Peach halves & slices | 10.0 | 10.0 |
| Pear halves & quarters | 11.0 | 11.0 |
| Pineapple cubes and rings | 12.0 | 12.0 |
| Raspberries | 7.0 | 7.0 |
| Strawberries | 9.0 | 9.0 |

| **FRUIT IN SYRUP (per 100g)** | | |
|---|---|---|
| Apricots | 18.0 | 18.0 |
| Black cherries | 17.0 | 17.0 |
| Fruit cocktail | 18.0 | 18.0 |
| Grapefruit segments | 18.0 | 18.0 |
| Mandarin oranges | 15.0 | 15.0 |
| Peach halves and slices | 16.0 | 16.0 |
| Pear halves and quarters | 17.0 | 17.0 |
| Pineapple cubes and rings | 18.0 | 18.0 |
| Prunes | 29.0 | 29.0 |
| Raspberries | 17.0 | 17.0 |
| Rhubarb | 14.0 | 14.0 |

| PRODUCT | CARBOHYDRATE (g) | SUGAR (g) |
|---|---|---|
| Rhubarb in light syrup | 8.5 | 8.5 |
| Strawberries | 18.0 | 18.0 |

**DRIED FRUIT**

| | | |
|---|---|---|
| Apricots, one | 3.0 | 3.0 |
| Raisins | 18.0 | 18.0 |
| Figs, one | 5.2 | 5.2 |
| Mixed dried fruit, 1 tbsp | 21.0 | 21.0 |
| Prunes, stewed, 6 | 6.0 | 6.0 |
| Sultanas, 1tbsp | 21.0 | 21.0 |

**FRESH FRUIT**

| | | |
|---|---|---|
| Eating apples | 12.0 | 12.0 |
| Banana | 23.0 | 21.0 |
| Blackcurrants, 100g | 21.0 | 21.0 |
| Black grapes, 50g | 13.0 | 13.0 |
| White grapes, 50g | 15.0 | 15.0 |
| Lemons | 0.6 | 0.6 |
| Mango, 2 slices | 6.0 | 6.0 |
| Melon, all types, one slice | 6.0 | 6.0 |
| Pineapple, 1 large slice | 8.0 | 8.0 |
| Raspberries, 20g | 3.0 | 3.0 |
| Strawberries, 20g | 6.0 | 6.0 |

**FRESH MEAT AND POULTRY contains no carbohydrates or sugars**

**MILK**

| | | |
|---|---|---|
| Evaporated milk, small can | 14.0 | 14.0 |
| Full-cream whole milk, ¼ litre | 14.0 | 14.0 |
| Healthy eating half-fat, ¼ litre | 14.0 | 14.0 |
| Virtually fat-free skimmed, ¼ litre | 15.0 | 15.0 |
| Soya milk, unsweetened, ¼ litre | 2.3 | 2.3 |

| PRODUCT | CARBOHYDRATE (g) | SUGAR (g) |
|---|---|---|
| **NUTS (per 100g)** | | |
| Dry roasted peanuts | 5.0 | 5.0 |
| Mixed nuts and raisins, small bag | 16.0 | 16.0 |
| Pistachios, 6 | 1.0 | 1.0 |
| Almonds, 6 | 1.0 | 1.0 |
| Walnuts, 6 | 0.7 | 0.5 |
| | | |
| **OFFAL contains no carbohydrates or sugars** | | |
| **OILS contains no carbohydrates or sugars** | | |
| | | |
| **PASTA (per 100g)** | | |
| Spaghetti | 51.0 | 2.0 |
| Macaroni | 68.0 | 2.0 |
| Pasta bows and shells | 68.0 | 2.0 |
| wholewheat lasagne and spaghetti | 62.0 | 4.0 |
| | | |
| **VEGETABLES** | | |
| Asparagus, 5 spears | 1.0 | 1.0 |
| Runner beans, 2 tbsp | 2.0 | 1.8 |
| Broccoli, 1 spear | 0.5 | 0.4 |
| Brussels sprouts, 2 tbsp | 3.0 | 2.7 |
| White cabbage, 1/6 | 4.0 | 4.0 |
| Carrots, 2 tbsp | 5.0 | 4.0 |
| Parsnip, 1 medium | 8.0 | 4.0 |
| Red pepper, ½ | 5.0 | 5.0 |
| Tomatoes, large tin | 6.0 | 6.0 |
| Yam | 43.0 | 9.0 |

## Proteins

All figures are rounded up or down to the nearest whole number in grams.

**PROTEIN (g) / PRODUCT**

**BREADS , CRACKERS AND CRISPBREADS**

| | |
|---|---|
| 7.0 | Bagel, 1 |
| 1.0 | Bread stick,1 |
| 4.0 | Chapati,1 |
| 1.0 | Cream cracker, 1 |
| 1.0 | Crispbread, 1 |
| 5.0 | Croissant, 1 |
| 3.0 | Crumpet, toasted, 1 |
| 4.0 | French bread, 5 cm pieces |
| 3.0 | Granary, 1 slice |
| 14.0 | Naan,1 |
| 1.00 | at cake, 1 |
| 2.0 | Poppadum, 1 |
| 7.0 | Pitta bread, 1 medium |
| 15.0 | Medium pizza |
| 4.0 | White soft roll, 1 |
| 4.0 | Wholemeal roll, 1 |
| 10.0 | Soda farl, 1 |
| 3.0 | Wheatmeal, 1 medium slice |
| 3.0 | White, 1 large slice |
| 3.0 | Wholemeal bread, 1 large slice |

**BREAKFAST CEREALS**

| | |
|---|---|
| 5.0 | All Bran, 40g |
| 5.0 | Alpen, 50g with sugar |
| 6.0 | Alpen, 40g, no sugar |
| 5.0 | Tropical Alpen, 50g |
| 3.0 | Bran Flakes, 40g |
| 2.0 | Coco Pops, 30g |
| 3.0 | Common Sense, 40g |
| 2.0 | Cornflakes, 30g |
| 3.0 | Country Store, 40g |
| 2.0 | Crunchy Nut, 40g |

**PRODUCTPROTEIN (g)**

| | |
|---|---|
| 2.0 | Frosties, 40g |
| 3.0 | Fruit n Fibre, 40g |
| 2.0 | Golden Grahams, 40g |
| 4.0 | Grape Nuts, 40g |
| 2.0 | Honey Nut loops, 50g |
| 5.0 | Swiss-style muesli, 50g |
| 2.0 | Cheerios, 40g |
| 4.0 | Porridge oats, 30g |
| 4.0 | Ready Brek, 30g |
| 2.0 | Rice Crispies, 30g |
| 5.0 | Shredded Wheat, 2 |
| 4.0 | Shreddies, 30g |
| 5.0 | Special K, 40g |
| 10.0 | Sugar Puffs, 20g |
| 4.0 | Sultana Bran, 40g |
| 4.0 | Sustain, 40 g |
| 4.0 | Weetabix, 2 |

## PROTEIN (g) / PRODUCT

### CHEESE

| | |
|---|---|
| 8.0 | Brie, average portion, 30g |
| 10.0 | Cheddar cheese, 30g |
| 12.0 | Low-fat Cheddar, 20g |
| 1.0 | Cream cheese (in sandwich) |
| 15.0 | Cottage cheese, small tub |
| 6.0 | Danish blue, 28g |
| 13.0 | Goats cheese, 1 individual |
| 10.0 | Mozzarella, 30g |
| 2.0 | Parmesan, 1 tbsp grated |
| 16.0 | Smoked, processed cheese, 30g |

### CREAMS AND MILK

| | |
|---|---|
| 0.5 | Double cream, 1 tbsp |
| 0.5 | Single cream, 1 tbsp |
| 2.0 | Condensed milk, 1 tbsp |
| 10.0 | Channel Island milk, 250ml |
| 9.0 | Full-fat cow's milk, 250ml |
| 10.0 | Semi-skimmed and skimmed, 250ml |
| 1.0 | Dried milk, 1 tsp |
| 14.0 | Evaporated milk, small can |
| 8.0 | Soya milk, 250ml |
| 13.0 | Greek yoghurt, 120g pot |
| 5.0 | Low-calorie yoghurt, 120g pot |
| 7.0 | Full-fat plain yoghurt, 120g pot |
| 6.0 | Low-fat plain yoghurt, 120g pot |
| 6.0 | Soya yoghurt, 120g pot |

### CAKES AND BISCUITS

| | |
|---|---|
| 2.0 | Battenburg, slice |

## PROTEIN (g) / PRODUCT

| | |
|---|---|
| 3.0 | Carrot and orange cake, slice |
| 6.0 | Chelsea bun |
| 0.71 | chocolate biscuit |
| 0.51 | chocolate chip cookie |
| 2.01 | cream horn |
| 6.0 | Danish pastry |
| 4.0 | Jam doughnut |
| 4.0 | Fresh cream eclair |
| 2.0 | Eccles cake |
| 3.0 | Fruit cake, 1 slice |
| 4.0 | Hot cross bun |
| 1.0 | 1 jam tart |
| 5.0 | Cheese scone |
| 2.0 | Swiss roll, slice |
| 4.0 | Cheesecake, 1 slice |
| 5.0 | Christmas pudding, average portion |
| 3.0 | Creme caramel |
| 3.0 | Ice cream, average portion |
| 4.0 | Lemon meringue pie, slice |
| 7.0 | Rice pudding, 1 small can |
| 6.0 | Trifle, portion |
| 1.0 | Lemon sorbet, 2 scoops |
| 4.0 | Suet pudding, portion |

### FISH

| | |
|---|---|
| 1.0 | 1 anchovy |
| 2.0 | Caviar, 1 tbsp |
| 29.0 | Cod in batter, 150g |
| 26.0 | Baked cod, 150g |
| 20.0 | Cod in parsley sauce, 150g |
| 25.0 | Crab, 1 dressed |
| 4.0 | 1 fish cake |

## PROTEIN (g) / PRODUCT

| | |
|---|---|
| 4.0 | 1 fish finger |
| 17.0 | Fish pie with potato, 150g |
| 28.0 | Smoked poached haddock, 150g |
| 37.0 | Grilled halibut, 150g |
| 15.0 | 1 rollmop herring |
| 34.0 | Boil-in-bag kippers, 170g |
| 28.0 | Smoked mackerel, 50g |
| 9.0 | 1 pilchard in tomato sauce |
| 27.0 | 1 plaice in breadcrumbs |
| 14.0 | Prawns, average portion |
| 20.0 | Tinned salmon, average portion |
| 24.0 | Fresh salmon steak |
| 14.0 | Smoked salmon, average portion |
| 13.06 | grilled sardines |
| 33.0 | 1 trout grilled |
| 25.0 | Fresh tuna, portion |

## MEALS WITH EGG

| | |
|---|---|
| 22.0 | Cheese omelette, 2 eggs |
| 6.0 | Poached egg |
| 23.0 | Quiche Lorraine, slice |
| 14.0 | Mushroom quiche, slice |
| 14.0 | Scotch egg |

## MEAT AND POULTRY

| | |
|---|---|
| 6.0 | Back bacon, grilled, 1 rasher |
| 5.0 | Streaky bacon, grilled, 1 rasher |
| 10.0 | Beefburger, grilled |
| 35.0 | Beef curry, average portion |

## PROTEIN (g) / PRODUCT

| | |
|---|---|
| 33.0 | Roast beef, 170g |
| 43.0 | Beef stir fry, average portion |
| 48.0 | Fillet steak, 170g |
| 53.0 | Sirloin steak, 170g |
| 45.0 | Rump steak, 200g |
| 25.0 | Roast chicken, 170g |
| 19.0 | Chicken leg |
| 32.0 | Chicken curry, average portion |
| 26.0 | Chicken Kiev, 1 |
| 19.0 | Chicken nuggets (6) |
| 12.0 | Chicken pie, individual |
| 31.0 | Chicken risotto, average portion |
| 96.0 | Tandoori chicken, average portion |
| 64.0 | Chicken vindaloo, average portion |
| 24.0 | Chilli con carne, average portion |
| 10.0 | Corned beef, average portion |
| 12.0 | Cornish pasty |
| 20.0 | Cottage pie, medium |
| 37.0 | Duck, roast, 170g |
| 47.0 | Gammon steak, average |
| 44.0 | Roast grouse, 1 whole |
| 6.0 | Ham, 1 slice |
| 33.0 | Kebab with pitta |
| 17.0 | Lamb chop |
| 24.0 | Roast leg lamb, 170g |
| 28.0 | Lamb biryani, average portion |
| 12.0 | Lamb's liver, 40g |
| 35.0 | Minced beef, lean, 150g |
| 28.0 | Moussaka, 200g |

## PROTEIN (g) / PRODUCT

60.0 Roast pheasant, 150g
39.0 Pork steak, grilled, 170g
27.0 Rabbit, quarter
14.0 Sausage roll
7.0 Low-fat sausage
15.0 Steak and kidney pie, individual
28.0 Turkey roast, 170g

## PULSES

7.0 Baked beans, portion
9.0 Broad beans, 2 tbsp
7.0 Butter beans, 2 tbsp
25.0 Chick peas, 2 tbsp
5.0 Kidney beans, 2 tbsp
3.0 Red lentils, 1 tbsp
4.0 Frozen peas, portion
11.0 Tofu, small cube

## BREAKFAST

50.0 Full English
50.0 Home-made kedgeree, 170g
30.0 McDonald's Big Break
20.0 McDonald's McLMuffin

## PROTEIN (g) / PRODUCT

20.0 Scrambled eggs on toast, 2 eggs
30.0 Smoked haddock, poached, 170g

## PUB FAVOURITES

30.0 Beef sandwiches, round
20.0 Cheese and pickle sandwiches, round
30.0 Cheese salad baguette
10.0 Crackers (4) and cheese
20.0 Crispbread (2), cottage cheese
10.0 Egg mayonnaise sandwiches, round
10.0 Hot dog, 1
20.0 Jacket potato, cheese
10.0 Jacket potato, plain
10.0 Pitta bread, houmous
10.0 Pitta bread, taramasalata
40.0 Ploughman's with Cheddar
10.0 Pork pie, individual
20.0 Prawn salad sandwich
30.0 Smoked mackerel salad

## Glycaemic Index

You need not become fixated with every detail of the glycaemic index (GI), but be aware that meals which are entirely high GI are not ideal for stable blood-sugar levels. An example would be a protein food such as meat or fish which is accompanied by potatoes, carrots, parsnips and swedes. This is the sort of meal which would have you falling asleep afterwards, especially if you also follow it with a heavy sweet pudding.

Try to mix high and low GI foods to give yourself an intermediate rating, and this will see you happily through in the short and the long term. For instance, rice pudding has the high GI rice together with the low GI milk, with a handful of dried fruit added for sweetness. Ideal low GI foods have one asterisk, intermediate GI foods have two.

| GI | BREADS AND BREAD PRODUCTS | GI | BREAKFAST CEREALS (30g servings) |
|----|---------------------------|----|----------------------------------|
| *20 | Pumpernickel, 1 piece | **42 | All Bran |
| **47 | Fruit loaf, 1 slice, 35g | **42 | Porridge |
| **55 | Honey and oat loaf, 1 slice | **44 | Muesli |
| **57 | Pitta bread, 1 piece | 55 | Special K |
| 60 | Hamburger bun | 57 | Bran Buds |
| 65 | Rye bread, 1 slice | 68 | Shredded Wheat |
| 68 | Croissant | 68 | Sustain |
| 68 | Crumpet | 68 | Weetabix |
| 69 | Ryvita, 2 | 77 | Coco Pops |
| 69 | Wholemeal, 1 slice | 80 | Puffed Wheat |
| 72 | Bagel | 82 | Rice Krispies |
| 70 | Melba toast, 4 pieces | 84 | Cornflakes |
| 70 | White, 1 slice | | |
| 90 | Gluten-free bread, 1 slice | | |
| 95 | French baguette, 1 slice | | |

| GI | FRUIT |
|---|---|
| *22 | Cherries, 80g |
| *25 | Grapefruit |
| *30 | Apricots, 6 dried, 30g |
| *30 | Peaches, tinned, portion |
| *38 | Apple |
| *40 | Apple juice, 250ml |
| *40 | Pear |
| *40 | Plums, 100g |
| **42 | Peach, fresh |
| **44 | Orange |
| **45 | Orange juice, 250ml |
| 45 | Grapes, green,100g |
| **52 | Kiwi fruit |
| **55 | Banana |
| **55 | Fruit cocktail, tinned, 125g |
| **55 | Mango,150g |
| **56 | Sultanas, 40g |
| **57 | Apricots, fresh, 100g |
| *64 | Raisins, 40g |
| 66 | Pineapple, 2 slices |
| 72 | Watermelon, slice |

| GI | DAIRY FOODS |
|---|---|
| *15 | Yoghurt, plain, low-fat, 120g pot |
| *27 | Milk, full fat, 250ml |
| *32 | Milk, skimmed, 250ml |
| *35 | Yoghurt, fruit, low-fat, 120g pot |
| **43 | Custard, portion |
| 60 | Ice cream, 2 scoops |

| GI | PASTA AND RICE (all cooked weight) |
|---|---|
| *35 | Vermicelli, 180g |
| *37 | Spaghetti, wholemeal, 180g |
| *40 | Spaghetti, white, 180g |
| 45 | Macaroni, 180g |
| 55 | Linguini, 180g |
| 55 | Semolina, 230g |
| 55 | Rice, brown, 100g |
| 55 | Popcorn, 30g |
| 58 | Rice, Basmati, 180g |
| 65 | Couscous, 100g |
| 68 | Gnocchi, 145g |
| 80 | Tapioca with milk, 250g |
| 87 | Rice, white, 180g |

| GI | PULSES (cooked per 100g) |
|---|---|
| *18 | Soya beans |
| *26 | Lentils, red |
| *27 | Kidney beans |
| *30 | Lentils, green or brown |
| *30 | Butter beans |
| *32 | Split peas |
| *38 | Haricot beans |
| **45 | Pinto beans |
| **48 | Baked beans |
| **50 | Kidney beans |

| GI | VEGETABLES |
|---|---|
| *22 | Peas, dried boiled, 70g |
| **48 | Peas, fresh, 80g |
| **54 | Potato crisps, 50g |
| **55 | Sweetcorn, 85g |
| *56 | Potato, boiled, 120g |
| 64 | Beetroot, 70g |

| GI | VEGETABLES (cont.) |
|---|---|
| 70 | Carrots, boiled, 70g |
| 70 | Potato, mashed,120g |
| 72 | Swede, 60g |
| 85 | Potato, baked,120g |
| 97 | Parsnips, boiled, 75g |

| GI | CHOCOLATE, BISCUITS, CAKES |
|---|---|
| ** 46 | Sponge cake, 1 slice |
| ** 47 | Fruit cake, 1 slice |
| ** 49 | Chocolate, milk,100g |
| 60 | Digestives, 2 |
| 64 | Shortbread biscuits, 2 |
| 65 | Fruit flan with pastry, 1 slice |
| 80 | Morning coffee, 3 |